Olympic Cookbook

50 HEALTHY RECIPES

from Ainsley Harriott and Team GB

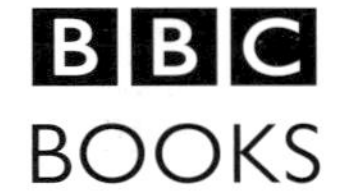

Jacqueline Boorman B.Sc. (Hons) SRD Accredited Sports Dietitian

Jacqueline Boorman has worked with the British Olympic Association (BOA) since 1997 when she became the consultant dietitian to the Olympic Medical Institute. In 1999 she was the BOA's HQ Nutritionist at the Gold Coast Training Camp, where athletes prepared for the Sydney Olympic Games, and she continues to be a member of the Sports Nutrition Advisory Group of the BOA. In addition to her work with the BOA, Jacqueline works with British Rowing, World Class Diving and UK Athletics and has worked with Oxford and Cambridge university rowing crews, the Royal Ballet, the London Contemporary Dance School and several professional footballers, golfers and boxers. She runs her own private practice based in London.

Published by BBC Books,
BBC Worldwide Limited, Woodlands,
80 Wood Lane, London W12 0TT

First published 2004

ISBN: 0 563 48788 7

Commissioning Editor: Nicky Ross
Project Editor: Rachel Copus
Cover Art Director: Pene Parker
Book Art Director: Sarah Ponder
Copy-editor: Deborah Savage
Designer: Susannah Good
Production Controller: Arlene Alexander
Food Stylist: Lorna Brash
Props Stylist: Penny Markham

Set in univers condensed
Printed and bound in Great Britain by The Bath Press
Colour origination by Radstock Reproductions Ltd, Midsomer Norton

All the spoon measurements in this book are level unless otherwise stated.
A tablespoon is 15 ml; a teaspoon is 5 ml. Follow one set of measurements when preparing any of the recipes.
Do not mix metric with imperial. All eggs used in the recipes are medium sized.
All vegetables should be peeled unless the recipe says otherwise.

contents

A word from Ainsley 4

Eating for health by Jacqueline Boorman 5

Breakfasts 12

Superfoods (Georgina Harland) 28

Light Bites 36

Carbohydrates (Sir Steve Redgrave) 48

Main Meals 60

Fats and oils (Linford Christie) 94

Desserts 108

Protein (Sharron Davies) 122

Index 128

A word from Ainsley

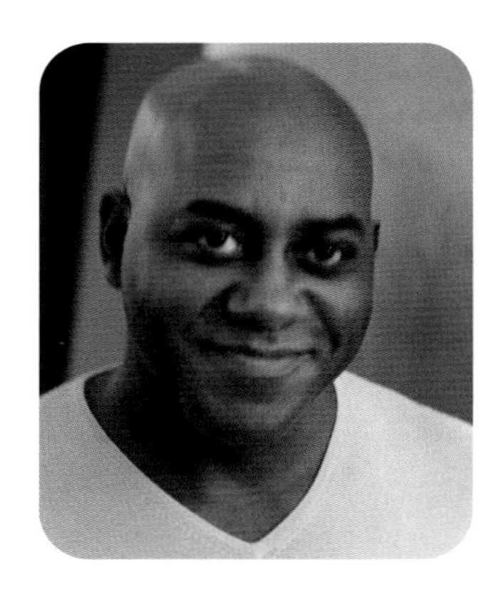

Buying this book won't turn you into an Olympian, or even the next Steve Redgrave or Denise Lewis! What I can guarantee, though, is delicious and healthy food without too much effort. We've even included some recipes from the athletes themselves.

But first we've got to wish the British Olympic Team lots of luck and look forward to seeing them compete at the highest level on the best stage in the world, the Olympic Games. It's always so exciting to see our Team GB at the Opening Ceremony, especially when you spot your favourite athlete. It's incredible to think that these few weeks are the climax of years of preparation for the athletes, both mental and physical, and a big part of their training is of course their diet. While the quantities of food that they consume are sometimes extreme (check out Steve Redgrave's food diary on page 48), one thing that they all have in common is they eat a rich and varied diet that keeps them in great shape for their sport. Throughout the book there are typical food diaries from several favourite British Olympians and I think you'll be amazed to see how much their diets vary depending on their sport.

I find that I'm constantly on the go with work, the kids, trying to keep fit and seeing friends. We're all busier now than ever before so it's vital that we look after our bodies and give them everything they need. So if you're worried that eating a healthy diet means cutting out all of your favourite foods, then think again. This book is all about giving you inspiration to eat well and live well. We've put together 50 great tasting recipes, all of which are guaranteed to do you good. As well as 40 brand new healthy eating recipes from me, ten of the UK's best -loved athletes have contributed their own favourite recipes to inspire you, including Sir Steve Redgrave, Audley Harrison and Sharron Davies. For a tasty breakfast treat, try *Honeyed Apricots with Vanilla Yoghurt*, or *Matthew Pinsent's Bacon-buster Sarnie*. Quick and easy lunch dishes include *Sweet Potato and Chick-pea Soup* and *Georgina Harland's Niçoise Salad*. How about some delectable choices from the Fish, Poultry, Meat or Vegetarian sections such as *Coconut Baked Fish with Papaya and Lime Salsa* or *Sizzling Beef in Black Bean Stir-fry*? There are also some fabulous desserts you can indulge in. Choose from *Blueberry Ripple*, *Sweet Rice Pudding with Mango and Lime* and *Sally Gunnell's Passion-fruit Water Ice* to name but a few.

I hope that you enjoy this book and that it will help you make the most of the wonderful fresh foods available. Once again let's wish the British Olympic Team lots of success and many gleaming medals dangling around their necks!

Happy Cooking!

Ainsley Harriott

Eating for health

by Jacqueline Boorman (consultant dietitian to The Olympic Medical Institute)

I have spent the last 15 years advising athletes of all shapes, sizes, backgrounds and disciplines about what they should eat and drink to improve their performance. During this time I have continued to see clients from all walks of life whose involvement in sport is on a more modest level or often confined to memories of their school PE lessons. It never ceases to amaze me that the similarities between these two disparate groups usually outnumber the differences. Indeed one common thread connects them all. That connection is that nothing, absolutely nothing, can replace a balanced diet.

Sports nutrition is a vast and multifaceted field and to try to condense it to give a brief overview without omitting any important information is an understandably difficult task. However, over the next few pages I will attempt to give a flavour of the discipline, and point to the areas of crossover from the advice I might offer an Olympian to the advice that is applicable to all of us.

Often it is the simple strategies that prove most effective in sports nutrition, for example: planning meals and snacks in advance; making a shopping list; keeping a food diary; and stocking up storecupboards with healthy foods. All of these have been used to great effect for the worn-out rower, the boxer needing to lose weight and the swimmer prone to throat infections, and they may well prove useful to you too.

Exploding the myths around sports nutrition

Myth 1

'Sports nutrition is about having special food and drink on the day of competition'

Granted, an athlete's consumption of food and drink on the day of competition will have some effect on their performance. However, sports nutrition is not a 'quick-fix' solution. Success in sport comes from weeks, months and years of hard work. It is the athlete's ability to recover both psychologically and physiologically from their day-to-day training that enables the athlete to push themselves to their limit. Aiming to eat sensibly every day is therefore vital both for elite performance and for day-to-day health.

Myth 2

'Sports nutrition is about nutritional pills and supplements that dramatically enhance performance'

Despite the media frenzy and hype surrounding supplements, there is very little evidence that athletes need extra vitamins and minerals if they are already eating a well-balanced diet. Taking pills as a short cut to eating well is never the answer and typically leads to illness, injury and unfulfilled dreams. The focus should always be on food and drink, not pills and potions.

why this book is important to you

The recipes in this book are derived from those used by top elite athletes during training and competition. However, it is just as applicable to everyone who leads a hectic and active life as it is to these elite few. Why? Because no matter whether we can run the 100m sub 10 seconds, or we are happy just taking the dog for a walk, we are likely to share some or all of the following four dietary goals.

1 **To manage our body weight successfully**
2 **To look after our immune system**
3 **To recover quickly from exercise**
4 **To maintain good energy levels**

After training, no sportsperson will want to spend hours shopping and cooking. They want quick, nutritious meals that enable them to meet their 4 goals. This is where knowledge about nutrition meets practice in the kitchen!

1 to manage our body weight successfully

Fat Most people who attempt to lose weight see fat as an enemy to be avoided at all costs. This is a mistake: our bodies do need some fat, but not at the expense of other important nutrients. However, you do need to remember that weight for weight fats and oils provide over twice the amount of calories as do protein or carbohydrate. In addition to this a high-saturated-fat diet could make you more at risk of heart disease or certain cancers. As a guide men and women, even if exercising, should consume the suggested daily amount of 95g and 70g fat respectively. Some suggestions to help achieve this might be:

> Enjoy smaller portions of meat, choosing lean cuts, removing the skin and trimming off visible fat.

> Go easy on butter, margarine, mayonnaise and dressings.

> Invest in a good non-stick pan and cook with less oil or fat. Use a pump-action oil spray which delivers a light coating of oil.

> Go easy on chocolate, crisps, rich desserts, cakes and biscuits. A chocolate bar and a packet of crisps could account for nearly 35g or half of a woman's daily suggested fat 'budget'!

Carbohydrate Concentrate on wholegrains such as wholemeal bread, brown rice, oats, whole-wheat breakfast cereal and pasta and starchy carbohydrates like potatoes and couscous for nutrient-rich fuels for hard-working muscles. Beans, lentils, most fruits and some vegetables are rich in slow-release carbohydrate. This means that blood sugars don't increase so rapidly after their consumption. Such carbohydrate-rich foods are more filling than refined carbohydrates, which is a bonus when watching your weight.

Timing (after 8pm!) It is a fallacy that you should not eat after 8pm for fear of it 'turning to fat'. It is how active you are and what you eat that will affect your weight, NOT the timing of your evening meal.

Portion size and balance
Managing your weight is all about the balance between calories consumed and calories burnt. Aim to have at least one third of your plate covered in vegetables or salad; the other two thirds with starchy carbohydrate or wholegrains plus meat, poultry or fish. If you are vegetarian, the remaining two thirds could be a mixture of grains and pulses.

Eating regularly Going long times without food may lead to rash and inappropriate food choices when the hunger pangs start. Don't do a panic food shop when you are hungry.

2 to look after our immune system

Following fad or quick-fix diets, crash dieting, heavy alcohol drinking and failing to eat regularly, particularly after intense exercise, will eventually result in your immune system suffering. A good variety of food, including at least five portions of fruit and vegetables each day, will go a long way to making you feel great. To say that one specific nutrient is more crucial than another would be to simplify a very complex bodily system; however, some nutrients have received more attention than others. These are some of the more important ones.

NUTRIENT	FOOD SOURCES
Vitamin C	Oranges, orange juice, potatoes, kiwi fruit, tinned tomatoes
Iron	Beef, lamb, pork, liver & liver pâté, salmon, tuna, greens, fortified breakfast cereal, wholemeal bread, nuts
Selenium	Brazil nuts, wholemeal bread
Calcium	Cows' milk, yoghurt, fromage frais, hard cheese, fortified soya milk, beans, almonds
Magnesium	Green vegetables, nuts, seeds, milk
Vitamin A	Cheese, eggs, full-fat milk and yoghurts, margarine, butter, mackerel
Zinc	Meat, poultry, fish, eggs
Water or fluids	Water, dilute juices, dilute squash

tip
For those training for more than 90 minutes at a go, a glucose-containing sports drink (30-60g of carbohydrate per hour) taken during exercise may help prevent them getting a cold.

3 to recover quickly from exercise

Fluids For daily health you should aim to drink approximately 8–10 large glasses or mugs of fluid every day and more is needed if you exercise. Precisely how much more is very individual, but the difference between pre- and post-workout weight can give a guide to how much you lose as sweat. Quick and complete rehydration after exercise requires you to consume a volume of fluid that is approximately 50 per cent greater than that which was lost as sweat: for example, if you lose 1kg (2.2lb) at the end of a session, you need to replace 1.5 litres (2⅔ pints) of fluid. Water and dilute juices are fine for light exercise, but to recover from intense exercise you might want to consider a sports drink or high-juice squash drinks and cordials.

A carbohydrate-rich snack Refuelling should start as soon as possible after exercise. A snack will be essential if your main meal is delayed. An excellent choice would be one that provided plenty of carbohydrate for refuelling muscles plus some protein to start repairing the body. Good combination snacks would be a banana milkshake, a yoghurt with some raisins, peanut butter on toast, or a bowl of cereal with milk. The size of the snack will depend on how hard you have worked out, the timing of your next meal and whether you are trying to control your weight.

Antioxidants Exercise is damaging – it produces substances called free radicals that can damage cells. But regular exercise 'trains' the body to cope with this damage and foods containing antioxidants may further protect you. Fruits and vegetables are rich in these antioxidants – not only because of the vitamins and minerals they contain such as vitamin C, beta-carotene and selenium, but also because of other naturally occurring chemicals such as their pigment. The vivid colours of foods such as carrots, mangoes, red peppers, blueberries and purple grapes demonstrate their ability to fight damage.

storecupboard saviours

Having the right ingredients to hand is the key to effortless cooking and it makes your time in the kitchen much easier. There are endless ways of using all those pastes, sauces and marinades. Use the list below as a guide to handy ingredients to keep in your storecupboard.

MINCED GINGER, GARLIC AND CHILLIES
Save on all that peeling, crushing and smelliness.

SOY SAUCE, HOISIN SAUCE, TERIYAKI SAUCE
Great for stir-fries.

PASTA, NOODLES, RICE, COUSCOUS
Great for bulking out dishes and a good source of carbohydrates.

DRIED FRUIT
Apricots, apple rings, mangoes, raisins and cranberries are all good low-fat snacks and good sources of iron and vitamin A.

CANNED MIXED PULSES, LENTILS, BEANS ETC.
Great sources of protein and carbohydrate and can be made very quickly into a simple but nutritionally balanced meal.

NUTS AND SEEDS
Generally good providers of iron, zinc, magnesium, essential fatty acids, Vitamin E and fibre.

OLIVE OIL
Healthier than butter!

SEASONINGS SUCH AS CAJUN OR CHICKEN
Rub into chicken pieces, drizzle with a little oil and bake for great-tasting chicken, hot or cold.

4 to maintain good energy levels

Although we have plenty of stored energy in the form of fat it is too slow a fuel to be solely used in vigorous exercise. It is carbohydrate that the body prefers to use when exercising intensely. So, strictly speaking, when you say, 'I've run out of energy,' it really means that your body has been unable to supply energy quickly enough to match its needs. The problem is that unlike fat, carbohydrate is stored in limited amounts in your liver and in muscles, and needs to be replaced before the next workout. Athletes, training every day therefore need to consume a higher-than-average carbohydrate intake to replace lost essential carbohydrate.

Carbohydrate: the amount

The amount of carbohydrate you need will depend on how much exercise you do and on its intensity, but we all need to include some wholegrain and starchy carbohydrates to achieve a diet where at least 50 per cent of our energy comes from carbohydrate. Endurance athletes like Matthew Pinsent need a high carbohydrate intake from bread, potatoes, pasta and rice but would also include refined sugars such as table sugar and glucose from sports drinks to cope with the rigours of training six hours a day. Of course he must still include wholegrains, good sources of protein-rich food and must not forget vegetables and fruit!

Carbohydrate: the type
Some types of carbohydrate affect blood glucose more quickly than others. This can be useful for athletes wishing to recover quickly. Fast carbohydrates include glucose sports drinks, jellybeans – even mashed potato! Some people prefer to base their carbohydrate intake around slow-release carbohydrates such as lentils, pasta, porridge, fruit and breads with 'bits' in such as pumpernickel bread.

Carbohydrate: the timing
Sources of carbohydrate should appear regularly in your diet through the day. Enjoying a carbohydrate-rich meal such as Vitality Pasta (page 101) after a hard workout is vital for recovery of muscle stores of glycogen (stored carbohydrate).

THE FOLLOWING COMPARES DAILY MEAL PLANS FOR A KEEP-FIT FAN AND AN OLYMPIAN

	EXERCISE GOAL: HEALTH AND/OR WEIGHT MANAGEMENT	EXERCISE GOAL: PERFORMANCE-RELATED
BREAKFAST	Breakfast Porridge made with low-fat milk. Fruit juice	Large bowl of porridge made with low-fat milk with chopped banana. Fruit juice
EXERCISE		Sports drink
MID-MORNING	Piece of fruit. Water, tea or coffee	Bowl of cereal with milk after exercise. Water, tea or coffee
LUNCH	Wholemeal pitta filled with mixed salad, diced chicken or houmous. Low-fat yoghurt. Fruit. Water, tea or coffee	Wholemeal pitta filled with mixed salad, diced chicken or houmous. Wholemeal toast and spread. Low-fat yoghurt. Fruit. High-juice fruit juice, water, tea or coffee
MID-AFTERNOON	Fruit or small cereal snack bar. Water, tea or coffee	Toasted bagel. Water, tea or coffee
EXERCISE	Water	Sports drink
SNACK	Water, tea or coffee	Milkshake after exercise
EVENING	Beef or cashew nut stir-fry with noodles. Water, tea or coffee	Beef/cashew nut stir-fry with extra noodles. High-juice fruit juice, water, tea or coffee
BEFORE BED	Low-fat milky drink	Low-fat milky drink. Wholemeal toast and spread

ten great britons

Amongst the recipes included in this book are ten provided by some of Britain's best-loved Olympians of all time. Although the sports with which they are involved are extremely diverse – from rowing to boxing to swimming – what they all share is a common concern for keeping themselves in peak condition. And, of course, that involves keeping a strict eye on their diet. Like the rest of us, though, all of the athletes here like to enjoy their food and so the recipes they have supplied are sure to make your mouth water. So, whether you're aim is just to feel a little more healthy, or if you've set your sights on becoming one of the next generation of great Britons, the advice given in this book should help set you on the right path. Between them, the contributing athletes have notched up an impressive 20 Olympic medals. Take a look at their biographies to find out more.

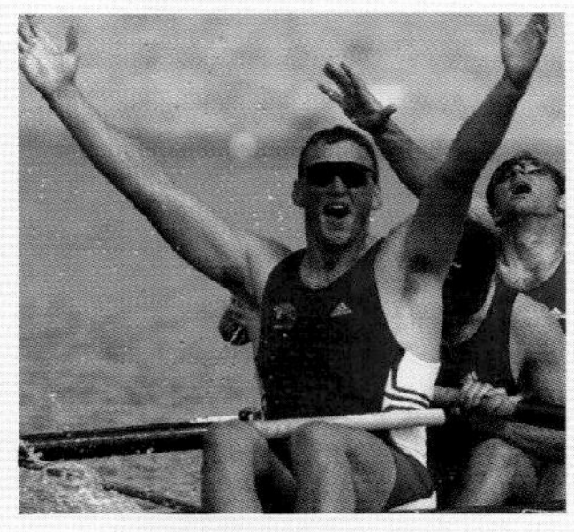

Matthew Pinsent

> **Olympics** Barcelona ('92), Atlanta ('96), Sydney (2000)

> **Medals** gold ('92), gold ('96), gold (2000)

> **Biography** Triple Olympic gold medallist Matthew Pinsent also holds ten world championship golds.

teamGB

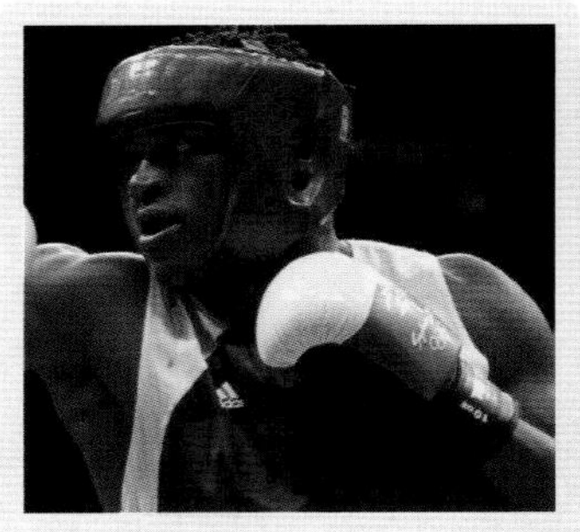

Audley Harrison

> **Olympics** Sydney (2000)

> **Medals** gold (2000)

> **Biography** Audley Harrison began his professional boxing career in 2001 after taking gold at the Sydney Olympics in 2000. He is now the reigning Olympic Super Heavyweight Champion.

teamGB

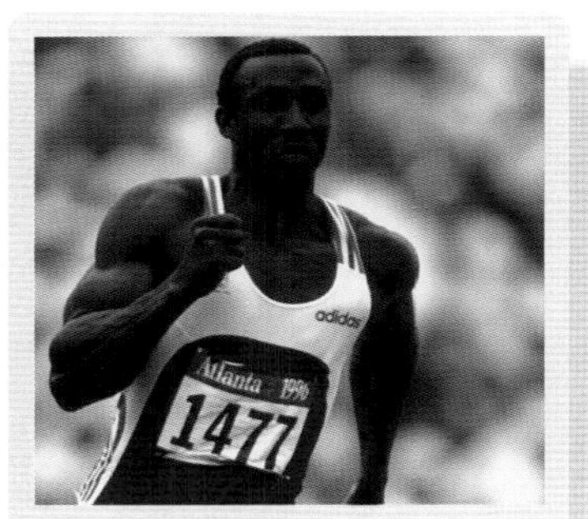

Linford Christie

> **Olympics** Seoul ('88), Barcelona ('92)

> **Medals** silver x 2 ('88), gold ('92)

> **Biography** Linford Christie was the first track athlete to hold the World, Olympic, European and Commonwealth titles at the same time. He retired from athletics in 1997.

teamGB

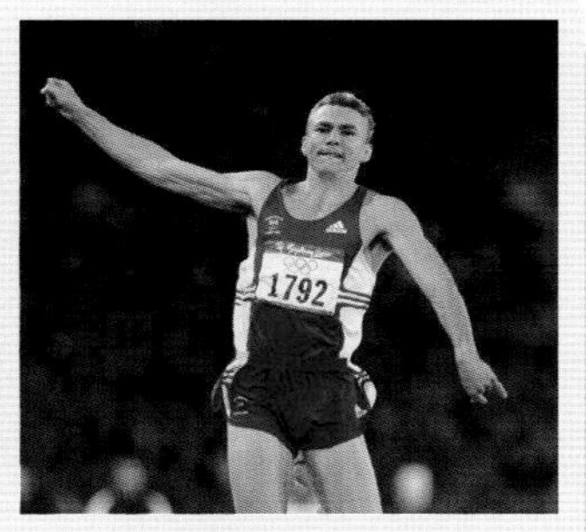

Jonathan Edwards

> **Olympics** Atlanta ('96), Sydney (2000)

> **Medals** silver ('96), gold (2000)

> **Biography** Triple jumper Jonathan Edwards retired in 2003. During the World Championships in 1995 he broke the world record twice on his way to a gold medal.

teamGB

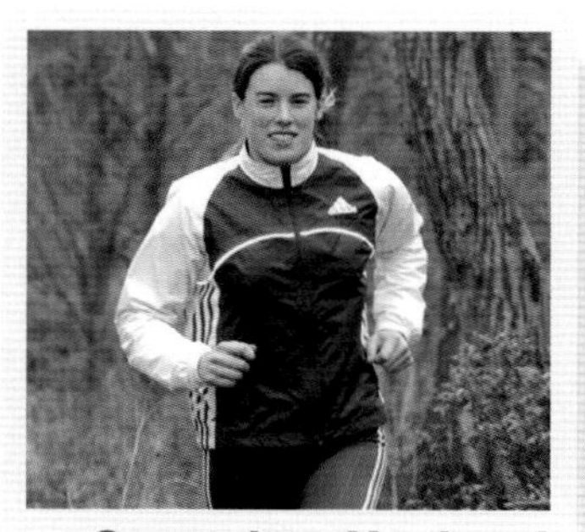

Georgina Harland

> **Biography** The 2004 Olympics will be the first Games for the 25-year-old modern pentathlete Georgina Harland. She won gold at the European Championships in 2003 – her first major international title.

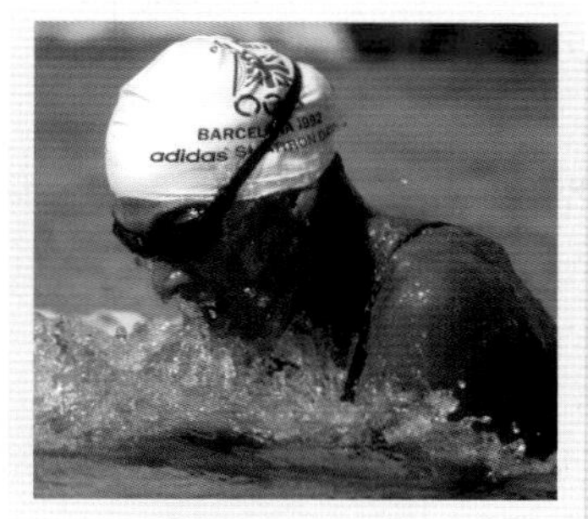

Sharron Davies

> **Olympics** Montreal ('76), Moscow ('80), Barcelona ('92)
> **Medals** silver ('80)
> **Biography** Sharron Davies burst on to the Olympic scene in 1976 at the age of just 13. She now combines charity work with a career in television.

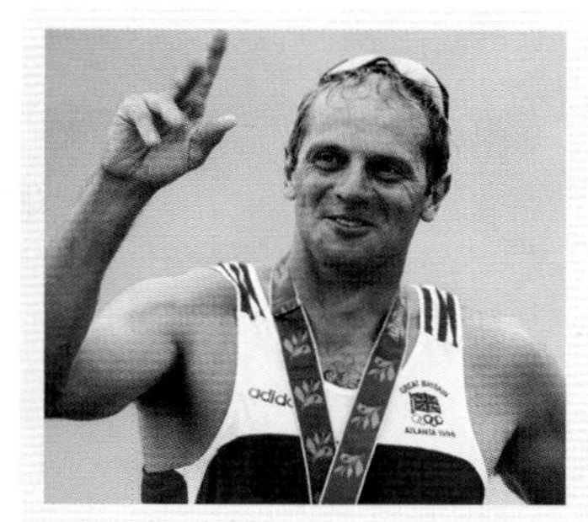

Sir Steve Redgrave

> **Olympics** LA ('84), Seoul ('88), Barcelona ('92), Atlanta ('96), Sydney (2000)
> **Medals** gold ('84), gold and bronze ('88) gold ('92), gold ('96), gold (2000)
> **Biography** The winner of five Olympic golds and nine world championships.

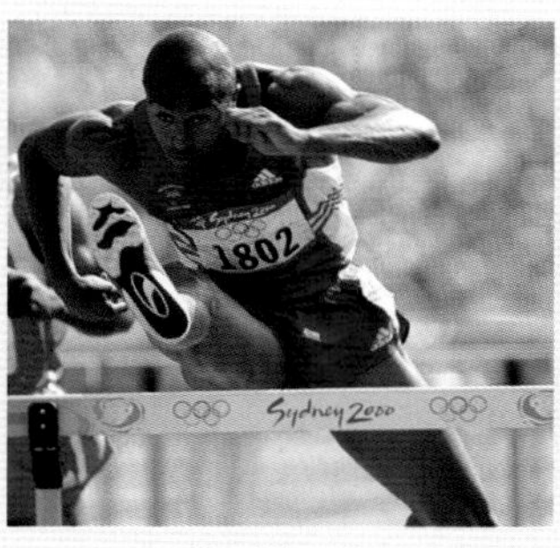

Colin Jackson

> **Olympics** Seoul ('88), Barcelona ('92), Atlanta ('96), Sydney (2000)
> **Medals** silver ('88)
> **Biography** During a career spanning 18 years, Colin achieved two world records and collected over 25 major championship medals.

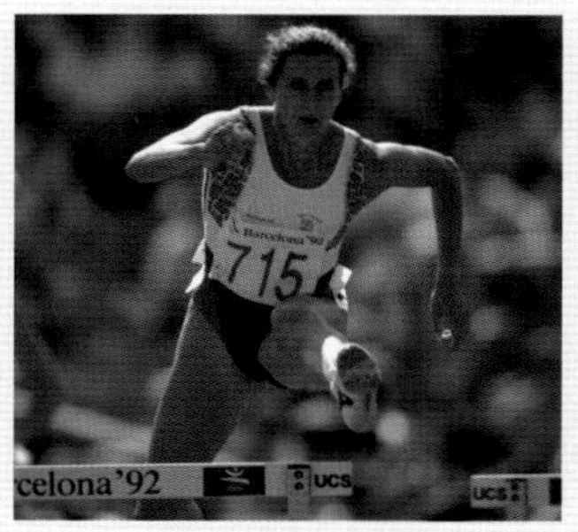

Sally Gunnell

> **Olympics** Seoul ('88), Barcelona ('92) Atlanta ('96)
> **Medals** gold and bronze ('92)
> **Biography** Sally Gunnell is the only woman to have held all four gold medals – Olympic, World, Commonwealth and European – at the same time.

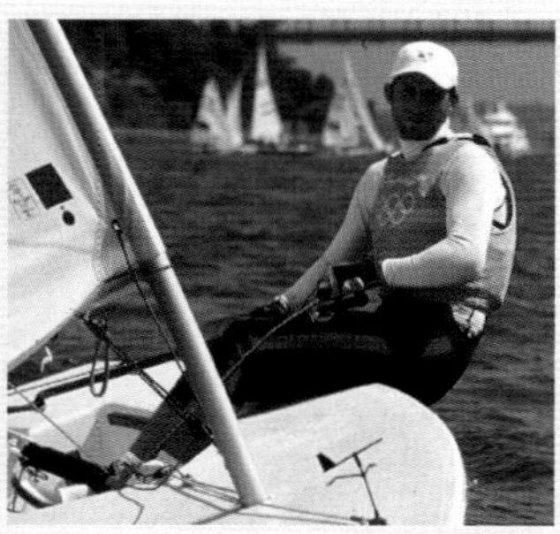

Ben Ainslie

> **Olympics** Atlanta ('96), Sydney (2000),
> **Medals** silver ('96), gold (2000)
> **Biography** Ben Ainslie was British Young Sailor of the Year in 1995. Since then he has competed for Britain at two Olympic Games, winning silver in Atlanta and gold in Sydney.

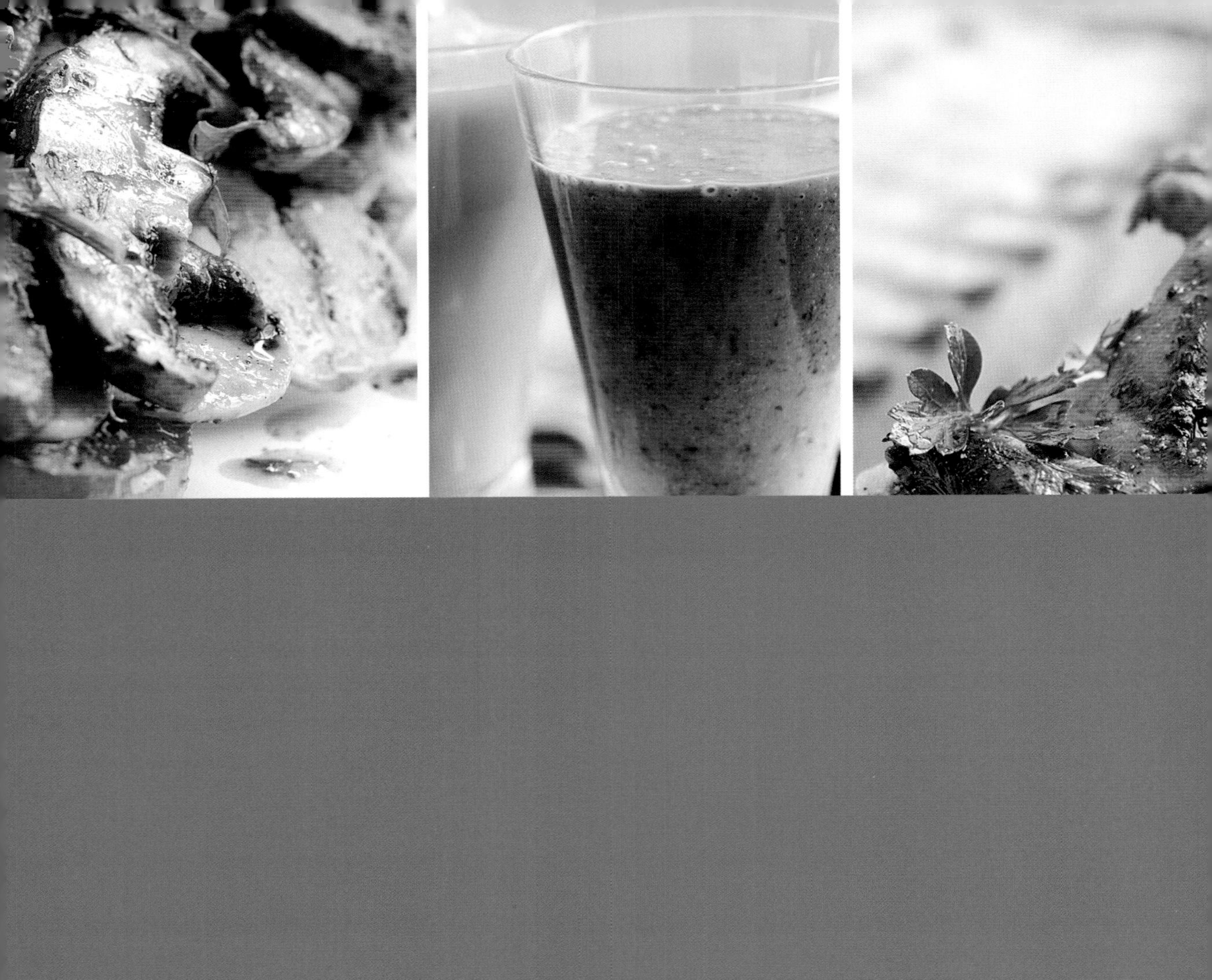

breakfasts

I'm sure you all get tired of hearing that breakfast is the most important meal of the day, but I have to say that it really is! And it's not just important for athletes – a good balanced breakfast will set body and mind up for the day ahead and you shouldn't feel tempted by sugary-fatty snacks later on. It doesn't have to be a boring slice of toast: have a go at some of these tasty brekkie suggestions – they're all delicious ... and good for you too.

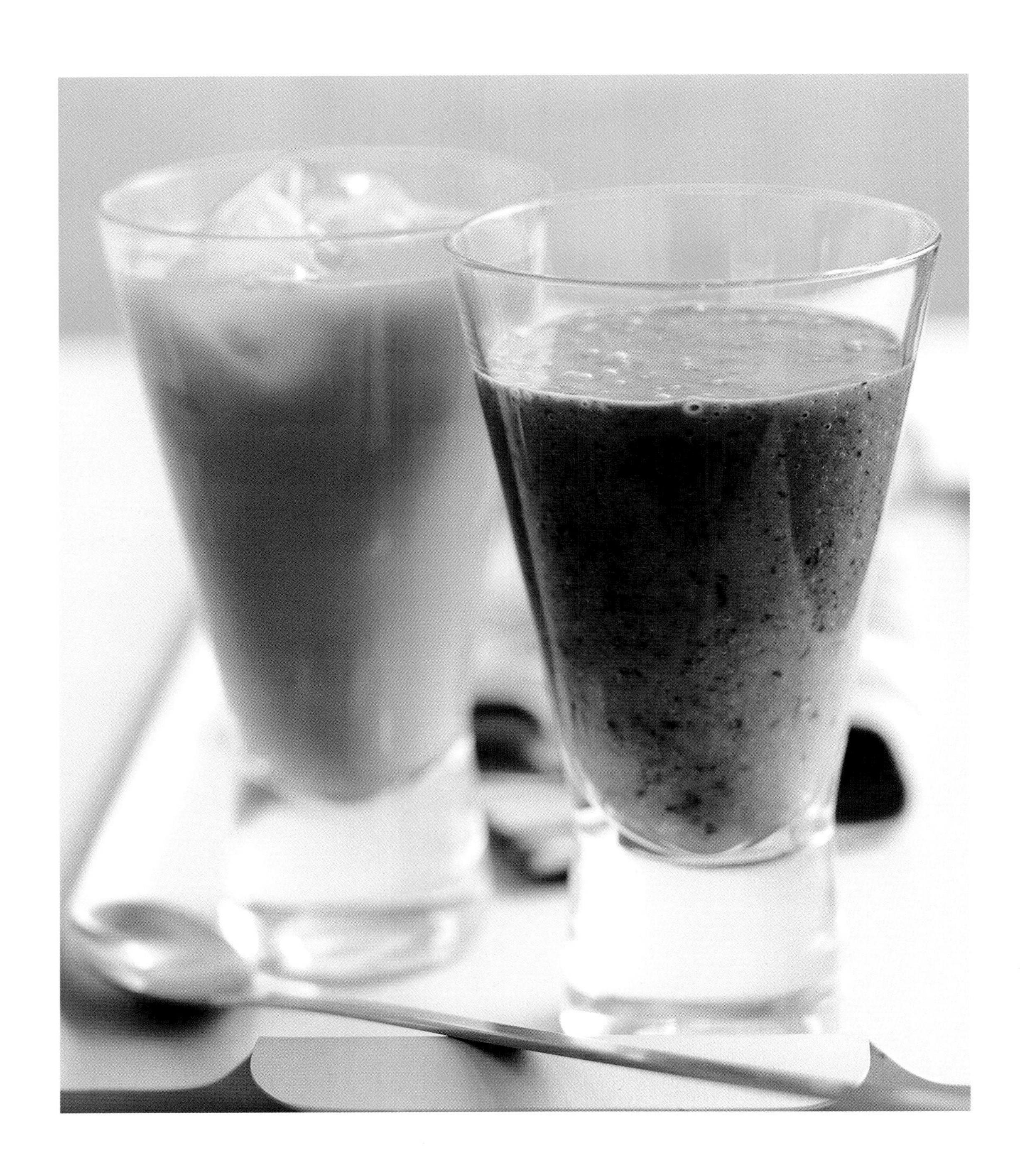

instant energy smoothies

We all know that fresh fruits and vegetables are good for us but not many of us would think of having them for breakfast. A simple juice can provide many of your essential vitamins and minerals for the day and all in one glass!

energy in a glass

3 carrots
2 apples, quartered
2.5 cm (1 in) piece of fresh root ginger
ice cubes, to serve

Preparation: under 5 minutes
Cooking time: none
Serves 1 (makes 350 ml/12 fl oz)

> Push all the fruit through the juicer, with the ginger, stir well. Put plenty of ice into a glass, pour in the juice and drink within 10 minutes to reap all the benefits.

nutritional information calories 194 • fat 1.3 g • saturated fat 0.1 g • added sugar none • fibre 10.2 g • protein 2.5 g • salt 0.2 g • carbohydrate 46 g

blue ribbon smoothie

juice of 1 lime
1 banana, peeled
100 g (4 oz) blueberries
2 scoops yellow-fruit frozen yoghurt
50 ml (2 fl oz) pure apple juice

Preparation: 5 minutes
Cooking time: none
Serves 1 (makes 350 ml/12 fl oz)

> Place all the ingredients in a blender or food processor and blend for 1 minute to a smooth thick drink.

nutritional information calories 254 • fat 1.4 g • saturated fat 0.6 g • added sugar 11 g • fibre 2.9 g • protein 6.9 g • salt 0.21 g • carbohydrate 57 g

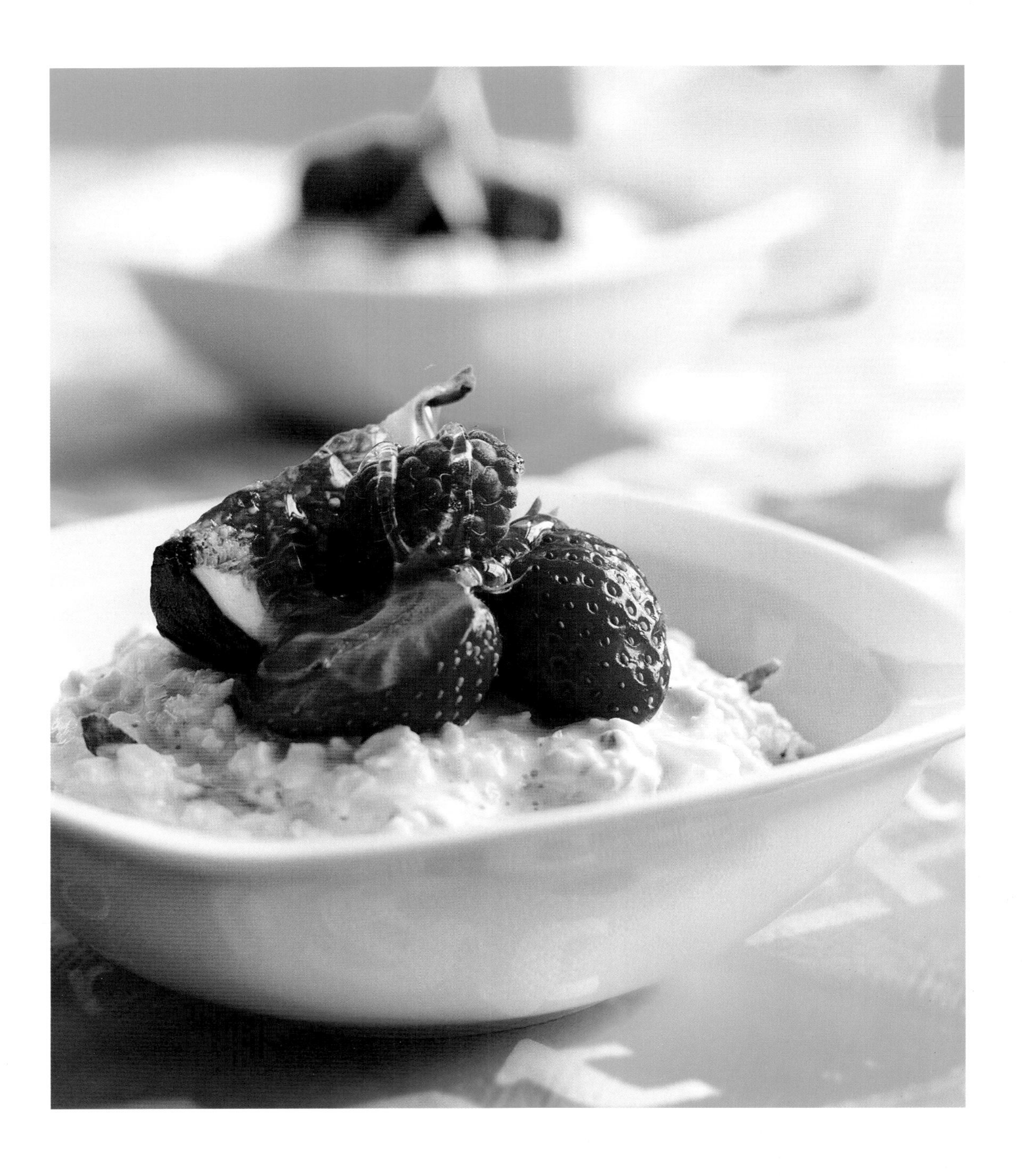

fresh fruit muesli

This muesli is exactly as the title tells you: 'fresh 'n' fruity'. It's the perfect way to start the day, with slow-release energy from the oats keeping you going right through till lunch. It's also a great healthy snack if you're feeling peckish between meals.

200 g (7 oz) jumbo rolled oats
225 ml (8 fl oz) apple juice
2 red-skinned sweet dessert apples
225 ml (8 fl oz) low-fat lemon yoghurt
juice of 1 lemon
2 tablespoons runny honey, plus extra to drizzle
1 fig, quartered
100 g (4 oz) mixed summer berries

Preparation: 10 minutes plus soaking
Cooking time: none
Serves 4

> Mix together the oats and apple juice, cover and leave to soak in the fridge for 1 hour or overnight.

> Peel, core and coarsely grate the apples and stir into the oat mixture with the lemon yoghurt and lemon juice. Sweeten to taste with the runny honey and spoon into serving bowls.

> Toss the fig with the mixed berries and pile on top of the muesli. Drizzle with extra honey to serve if liked.

nutritional information calories 336 • fat 4.1 g • saturated fat 1 g • added sugar 13.2 g • fibre 7.3 g • protein 11.2 g • salt 0.11 g • carbohydrate 68 g

honeyed apricots with vanilla yoghurt

All fruits, including dried ones, are an instant source of energy. The dried apricots used in this recipe are rich in iron and vitamin A but you can use whatever your favourite fruits are – fresh or dried fruit is an excellent source of fibre.

175 g (6 oz) dried apricots
300 ml (½ pint) orange juice
1 large vanilla pod
500 g (1 lb 2 oz) tub of 0%-fat Greek-style yoghurt
3 tablespoons runny honey
25 g (1 oz) flaked almonds, toasted
2 teaspoons sesame seeds, toasted

Preparation: 15 minutes
Cooking time: 20–25 minutes
Serves 4

> Place the dried apricots, orange juice and vanilla pod in a saucepan, bring to the boil and then simmer, uncovered, for 20–25 minutes. Leave to cool completely.

> Remove the vanilla pod, scrape out the seeds and stir them into the yoghurt. Spoon the apricot mixture into four individual serving glasses and drizzle over the runny honey. Spoon over the yoghurt mixture. Sprinkle with the nuts and seeds. Serve immediately.

nutritional information calories 259 • fat 5 g • saturated fat 0.4 g • added sugar 8.6 g • fibre 4.1 g • protein 16.8 g • salt 0.3 g • carbohydrate 39 g

healthy eating

> We all need iron for healthy blood and immune systems, and children in particular require iron-rich foods while they grow. Why not keep a bag of dried apricots in the cupboard and hand them out to hungry children between meals as an alternative to sweets or biscuits?

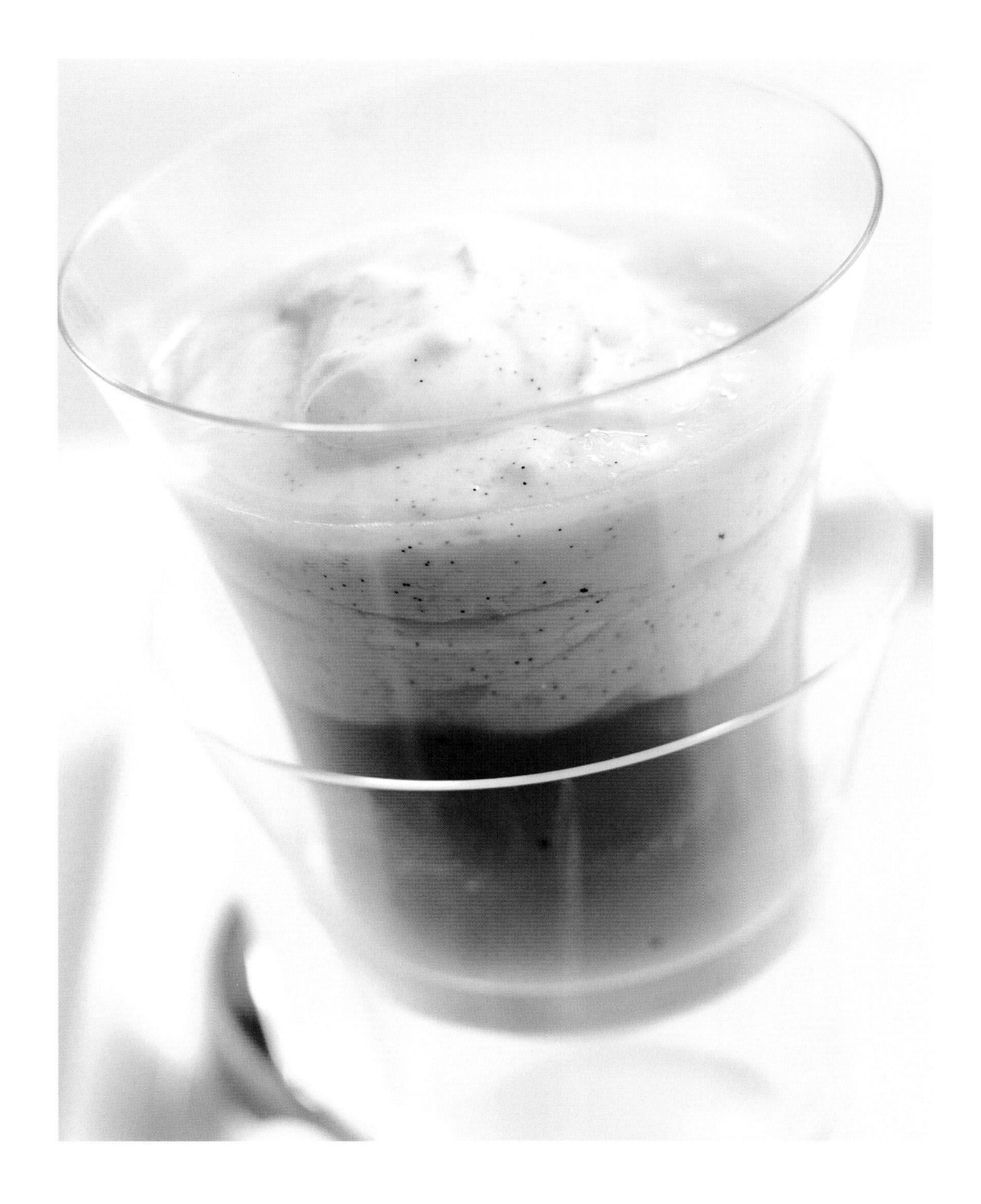

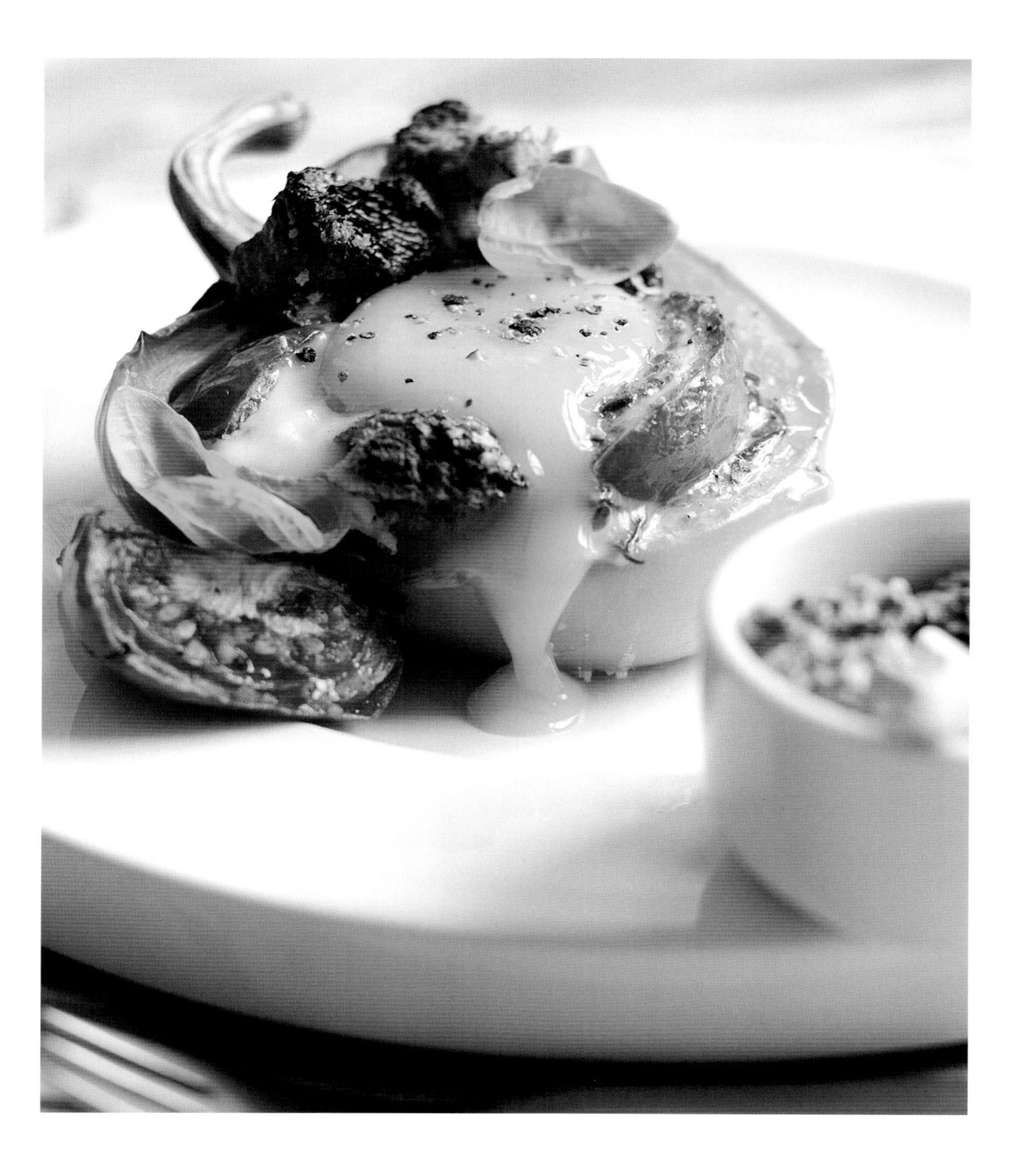

pepper and egg sauté

Many vegetables make great containers for tasty stuffings and peppers are no exception. You could oven-bake a few sausages when you roast the peppers or add a slice of chopped bacon to the filling.

- 1 slice of wholemeal toast
- 1 large field mushroom, cut into chunks
- 2 ripe tomatoes, cut into wedges
- small handful of basil leaves, plus extra to garnish
- 1 tablespoon olive oil
- 1 yellow pepper, halved and seeded
- 1 orange pepper, halved and seeded
- 4 medium eggs
- salt and freshly ground black pepper

Preparation: 15 minutes
Cooking time: 25–30 minutes
Serves 4

> Preheat the oven to 200°C/400°F/Gas Mark 6. Tear the wholemeal toast into small pieces and place in a bowl with the mushrooms, tomatoes, basil and olive oil. Season with salt and freshly ground black pepper and toss well to combine. Spoon the mixture into the pepper halves and place in a small roasting tin. Roast for 20 minutes.

> Make four hollows in the vegetable mixture with the back of a spoon, pushing the filling up the sides of the peppers to create a wall. Crack an egg into each one and return to the oven for 5–7 minutes until the egg is set or cooked to your liking. Sprinkle over the extra basil to garnish and season well. Serve with crusty bread.

nutritional information calories 142 • fat 8.7 g • saturated fat 2 g • added sugar none • fibre 1.9 g • protein 8.5 g • salt 0.59 g • carbohydrate 8 g

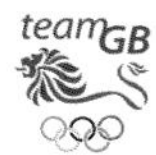

Matthew Pinsent's

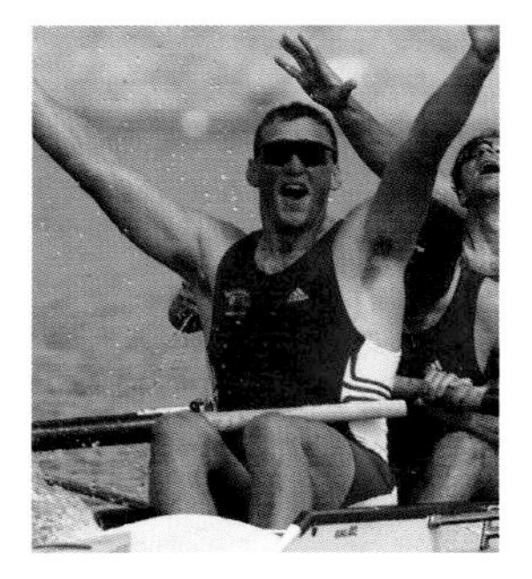

bacon-buster sarnie

Bread contains masses of carbohydrate energy and hardly any fat. Choose your favourite roll – wholemeal is better but ciabatta and panini toast so well on the griddle. Turkey rashers are a great alternative to bacon as they are lower in fat.

1 half ciabatta loaf or 1 panini roll or 1 soft wholemeal sub roll, split in half
1 tablespoon olive oil
1 beefsteak tomato, thickly sliced
2 Portabello mushrooms, thickly sliced
2 tablespoons chopped parsley, plus extra to garnish
3 unsmoked turkey rashers
2 tablespoons tomato ketchup (optional)
salt and freshly ground black pepper

Preparation: 10 minutes
Cooking time: 8 minutes
Serves 1

> Brush the ciabatta, panini or wholemeal roll with a little of the oil.

> Toss together the remaining oil, tomato and mushroom slices and parsley and season well with salt and pepper.

> Heat a large griddle pan until hot and smoking and place the bread, crust-side down, on the griddle. Press down well with a fish slice or the base of another pan and hold down for 2–3 minutes until toasted and charred with lines. Remove and wrap in a clean cloth to keep warm.

> Tip the vegetables on to one side of the griddle. Arrange the turkey rashers on the other side of the griddle and cook both for 2–3 minutes or until the rashers are golden, turning them over once during cooking.

> Pile the vegetables on to the bottom half of the bread, top with the turkey rashers and spoon over the tomato ketchup, if using. Scatter over the remaining parsley. Sandwich with the other half of the bread, press down well and eat immediately!

nutritional information calories 524 • fat 16.7 g • saturated fat 2.9 g • added sugar 1.8 g • fibre 6.5 g • protein 28.6 g • salt 5.8 g • carbohydrate 65 g

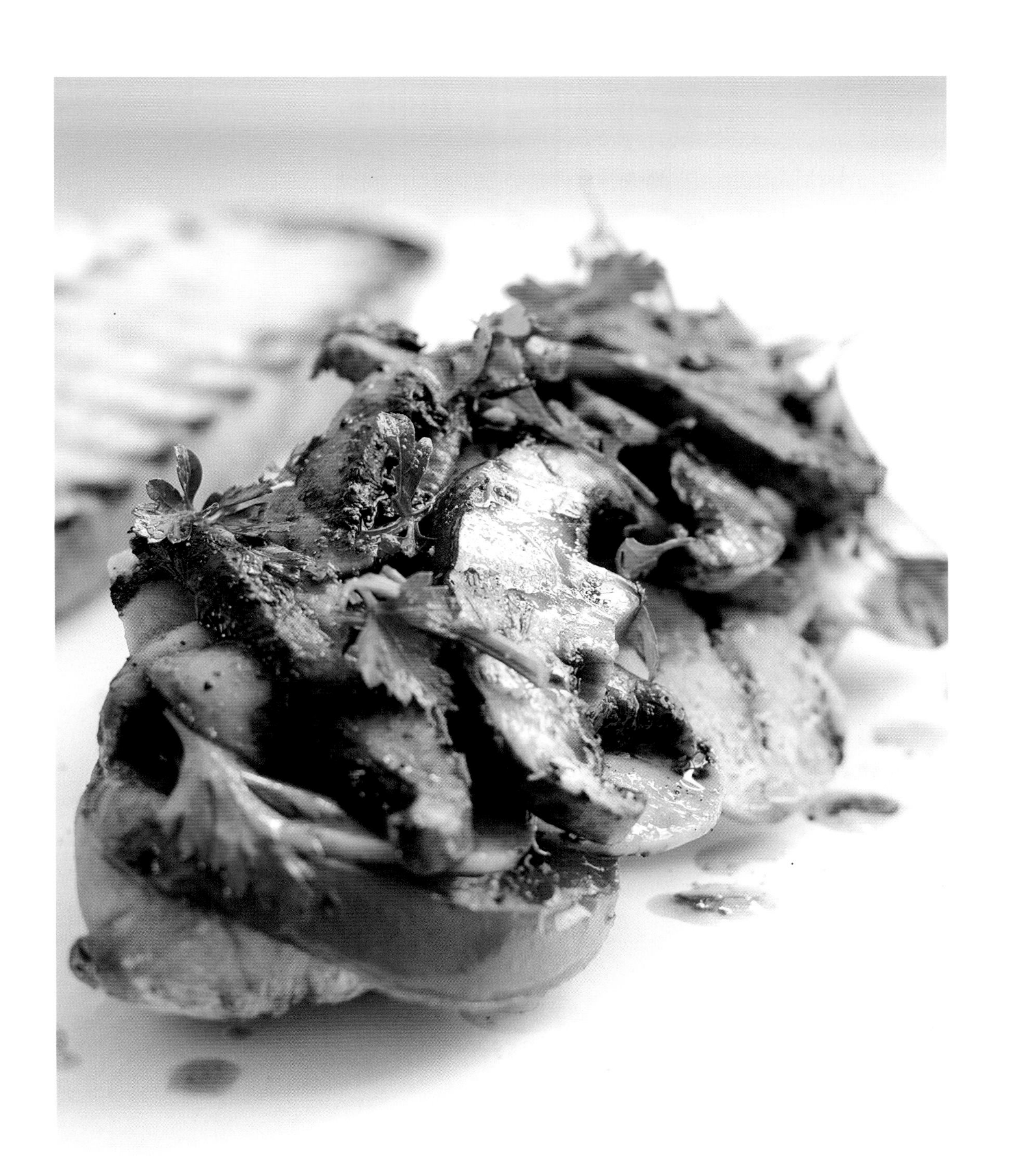

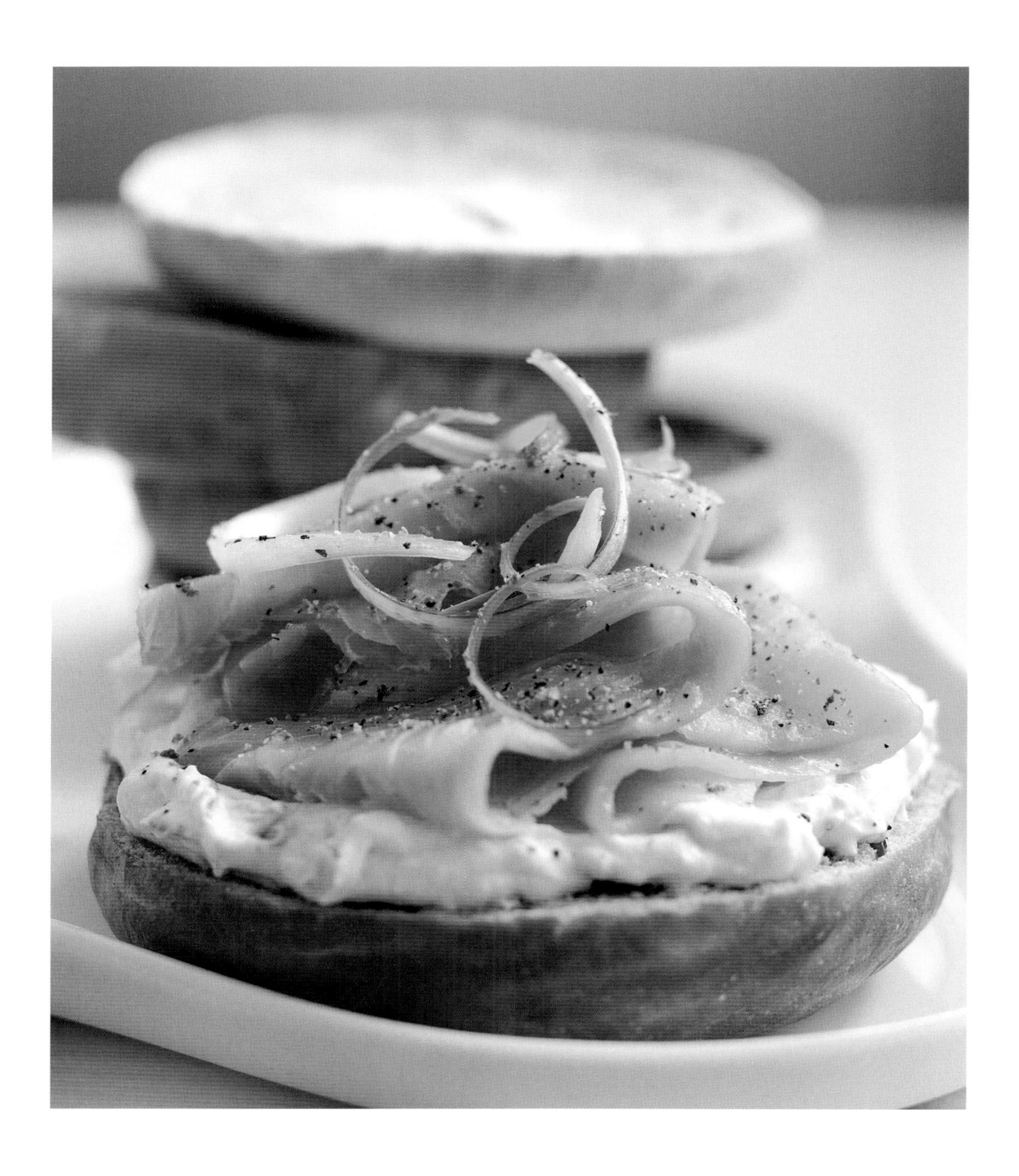

hot salmon bagel

Quark is a great low-fat alternative to cream cheese, with only 0.2 g fat per 100 g. Mix it with smoked salmon and you get a lovely cheat's version of a classic, great-tasting breakfast, brunch or snack.

250 g tub of quark (semi-skimmed-milk soft cheese)
juice and finely grated zest of ½ small lemon
1 tablespoon horseradish sauce
4 spring onions, trimmed
2 plain bagels, halved
175 g (6 oz) smoked salmon
freshly ground black pepper
lemon wedges, to serve

Preparation: 10–15 minutes
Cooking time: 2–3 minutes
Serves 4

> Mix together the quark, lemon zest and juice and horseradish until smooth and creamy. Season to taste with freshly ground black pepper.

> Finely chop three of the spring onions and stir into the cheese mixture. Finely shred the remaining spring onion and place in a bowl of cold water for 5 minutes.

> Toast the bagels until golden. Spread with the cheese mixture. Arrange the smoked salmon over the cheese mixture. Drain the spring onion and scatter over the smoked salmon. Season with plenty more pepper and serve with lemon wedges to squeeze over.

nutritional information calories 203 • fat 3 g • saturated fat 0.5 g • added sugar 0.3 g • fibre 1.1 g • protein 23.9 g • salt 2.9 g • carbohydrate 21 g

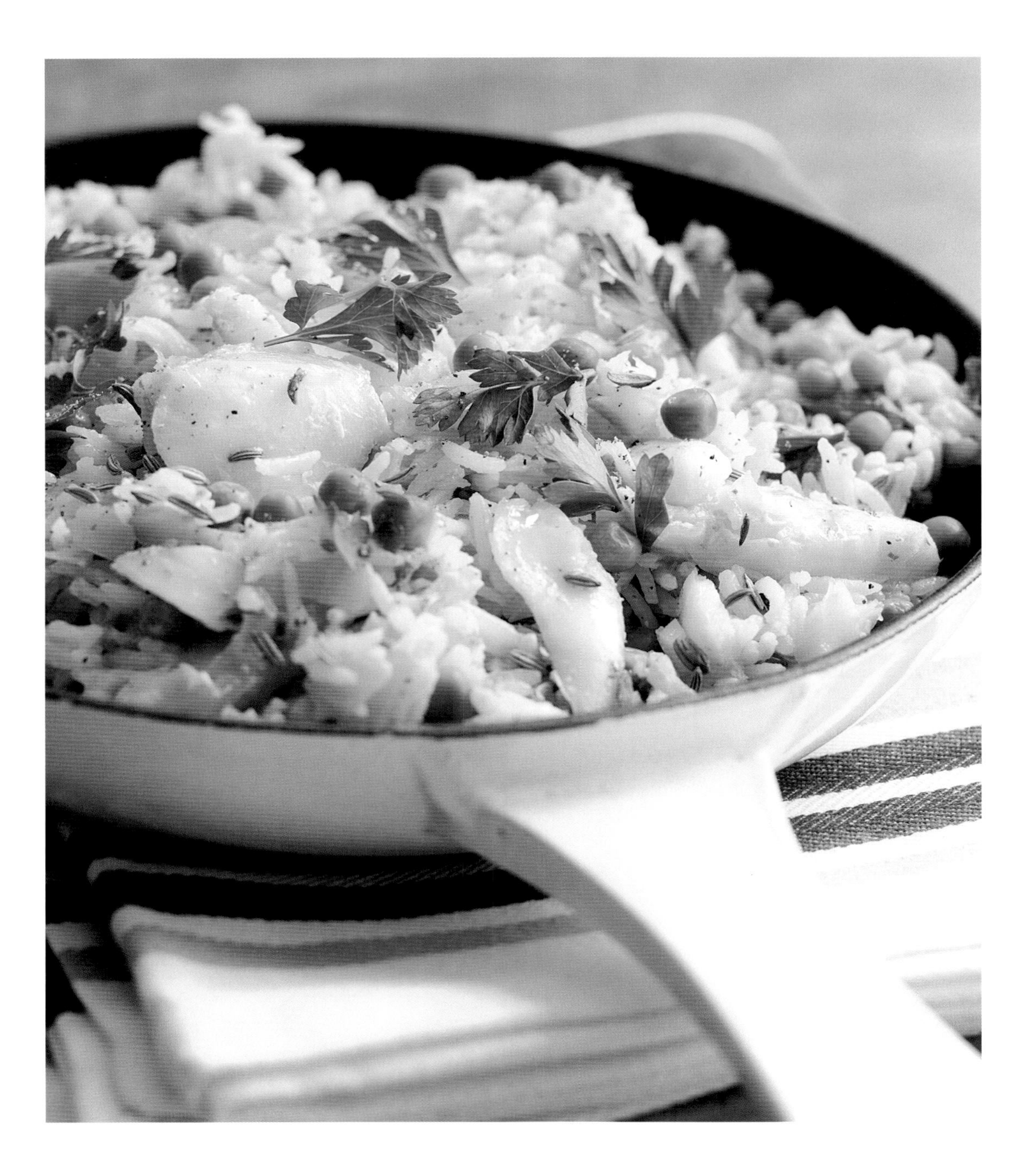

one-pan, one-cook kedgeree

Served for breakfast in colonial India and still enjoyed today – you can't beat kedgeree on a cold winter's morning. Like most fish, smoked haddock is a good, low-fat, low-calorie source of protein. Combined with rice it gives you a great energy-boosting start to the day.

- 2 teaspoons olive oil
- 1 large onion, finely chopped
- 2 teaspoons fennel seeds, crushed
- 300 g (10 oz) basmati rice
- 175 g (6 oz) frozen peas
- 1 teaspoon salt
- 450 g (1 lb) smoked haddock, skinned
- 3 tablespoons half-fat crème fraîche
- salt and freshly ground black pepper
- small handful of chopped parsley, to garnish

Preparation: 15 minutes
Cooking time: 20 minutes
Serves 4

> Heat the oil in a medium-sized saucepan and fry the onion and fennel seeds for 3–4 minutes, until the onion has softened.

> Add the rice, peas and salt and pour over 700 ml (1¼ pints) of water. Lay the fish on top. Bring to the boil, cover and simmer for 14–15 minutes on the lowest heat possible, until all the liquid has been absorbed.

> Remove the lid and flake the fish with a fork. Stir in the crème fraîche and season to taste. Scatter over the parsley before serving.

nutritional information calories 428 • fat 5.1 g • saturated fat 1.6 g • added sugar none • fibre 2.9 g • protein 30.8 g • salt 3.71 g • carbohydrate 69 g

healthy eating

> By using half-fat crème fraîche, you cut down on the number of calories from fat, but don't lose out on flavour!

“I drink squash all day and isotonic drinks in some training sessions. For snacks in between training I would choose malt loaf, wholemeal toast and home-made marmalade.” > **Georgina Harland**

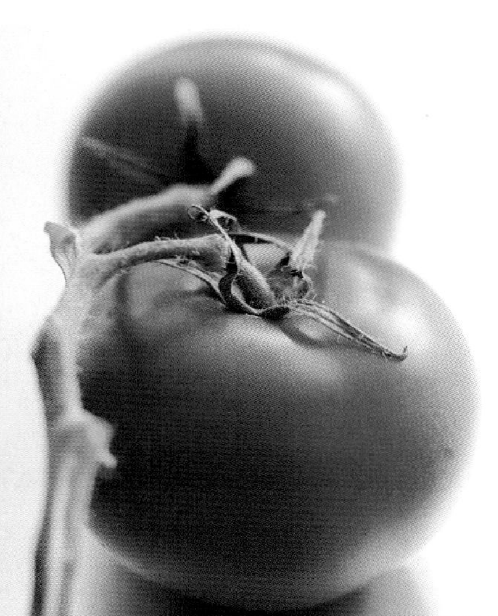

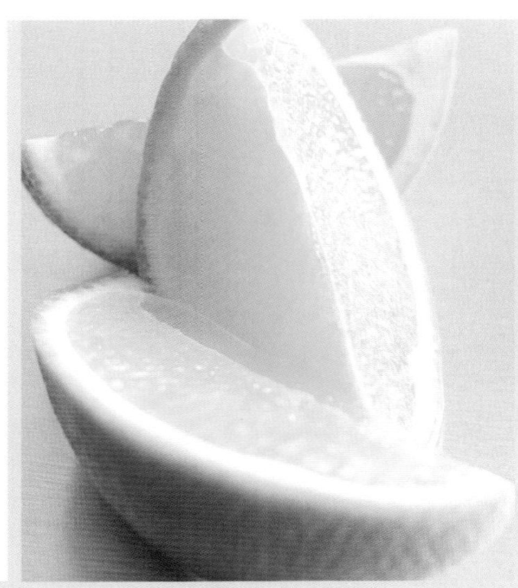

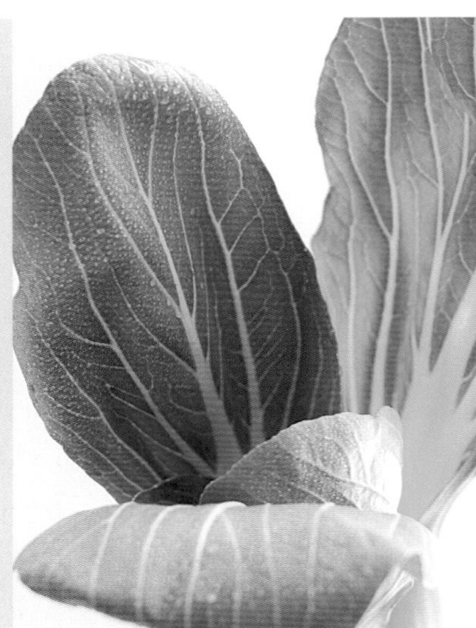

FOOD	NUTRIENTS OR PHYTOCHEMICALS
Olives and olive oil	vitamin E, antioxidant phytochemicals
Orange juice	vitamin C, potassium
Tomatoes	vitamins C and E, carotenoids, antioxidant lycopene (when cooked)
Parsley	iron and vitamin C
Dried apricots and mangoes	iron, fibre, potassium, vitamin C, antioxidant beta-carotene
Grapes	potassium, antioxidant phytochemicals
Home-made orange marmalade	antioxidant phytochemicals, pectin
Nuts and seeds found in breakfast cereal and muesli bars	iron, zinc, copper, magnesium, potassium, vitamins B1 and E, antioxidant phytochemicals
Tea	antioxidant phytochemicals

It is not just the carbohydrates for fuel, protein for repair and essential fats for health that are on the mind of Britain's number 1 modern pentathlete – she also has to consider the vitamins, minerals and phytochemicals found in foods. Phytochemicals are a group of compounds that occur naturally in foods such as fruit, vegetables, nuts, seeds and wholegrains. They are thought to offer some

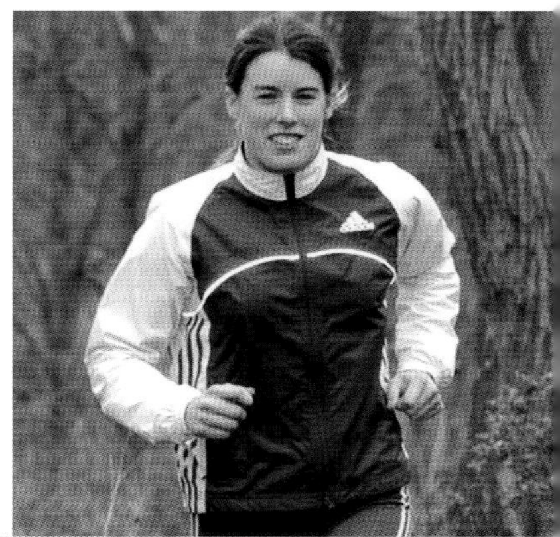

superfoods

protection against conditions such as cancer and heart disease. The term 'superfoods' has been coined to describe foods that are super sources of vitamins, minerals and antioxidants. These superfoods are vital for top athletes who wish to optimise health and performance. A lack of fruit and vegetables would create a very unbalanced diet, where an athlete would be prone to infections, show poor recovery and repair after training. Such athletes would need to rely heavily on supplements – something that is undersirable as supplements can never completely replace the hundreds of antioxidants found in a well-balanced diet. Athletes need to eat at least five portions of fruit and vegetables a day. Remember, a portion could be any of the following:

- 1 medium fruit, such as apple, orange, banana
- 2–3 tablespoons fresh fruit salad, stewed or canned fruit
- 150 ml (¼ pint) glass fruit juice
- 2 tablespoons vegetables (raw or cooked, fresh, frozen or canned)
- 1 dessert-bowlful salad
- 1 tablespoon dried fruit, such as raisins

The modern pentathlon requires Georgina to be proficient in five disciplines: swimming; running; air-pistol shooting; fencing and show jumping. Despite having a hectic training schedule and having to 'eat on the hop', Georgina plans balanced meals and superfood snacks. A look at her diet reveals the superfoods shown in the table, left.

Georgina's food diary

> **Breakfast before training**

Bowl of muesli or oat cluster with fruit
Semi-skimmed milk
Glass of apple juice.

> **Lunch**

2 rounds of wholemeal-bread sandwiches (no butter or mayonnaise) filled with ham or tuna and salad
or niçoise salad (see recipe, page 56) with wholemeal bread
Fruit such as grapes and chocolate.

> **Main Meal**

Always some pasta, rice or potatoes
Chicken stir-fry with lots of vegetables and rice
Red meat at least once a week: for example, bolognese sauce or pork chop
Followed by a yoghurt for calcium.

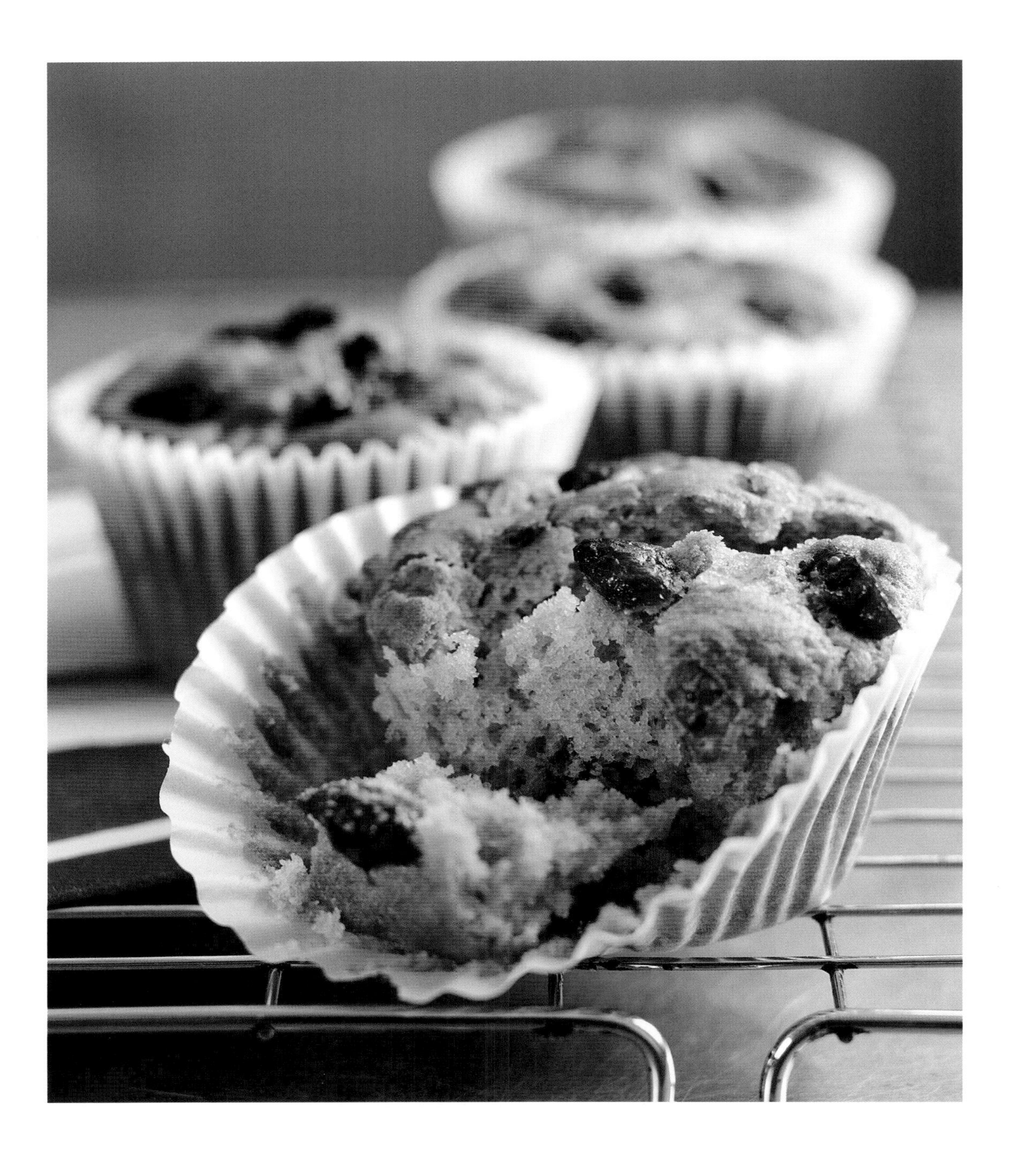

figgy muffins

These tasty muffins are great to grab on the way out of the door if you are in a rush and haven't got time to sit down for breakfast. A great source of beta-carotene, iron and potassium, and fibre which helps digestion.

225 g (8 oz) self-raising flour
1 tablespoon baking powder
3 tablespoons light muscovado sugar
175 g (6 oz) dried figs, roughly chopped
2 medium eggs, beaten
150 ml (¼ pint) semi-skimmed milk
3 tablespoons vegetable oil
50 g (2 oz) crystallised coffee-sugar granules (optional)

Preparation: 20 minutes
Cooking time: 20–25 minutes
Makes 12

> Preheat the oven to 200°C/400°F/Gas Mark 6. Line 12 holes of a muffin tin with deep paper cases. Sift the flour and baking powder together into a large mixing bowl. Stir in the sugar and 125 g (4 oz) of the figs.

> Beat together the eggs, milk and oil in a measuring jug. Pour over the flour mixture and, using a large metal spoon, fold the liquid into the dry mixture until the two are just mixed. Don't be tempted to over mix – it should look slightly lumpy.

> Spoon the mixture into the muffin cases. Sprinkle over the remaining figs and the sugar granules, if using. Bake for 20–25 minutes until the muffins are risen and golden.

nutritional information calories 154 • fat 4.3 g • saturated fat 0.9 g • added sugar 3.8 g • fibre 1.7 g • protein 3.7 g • salt 0.62 g • carbohydrate 27 g

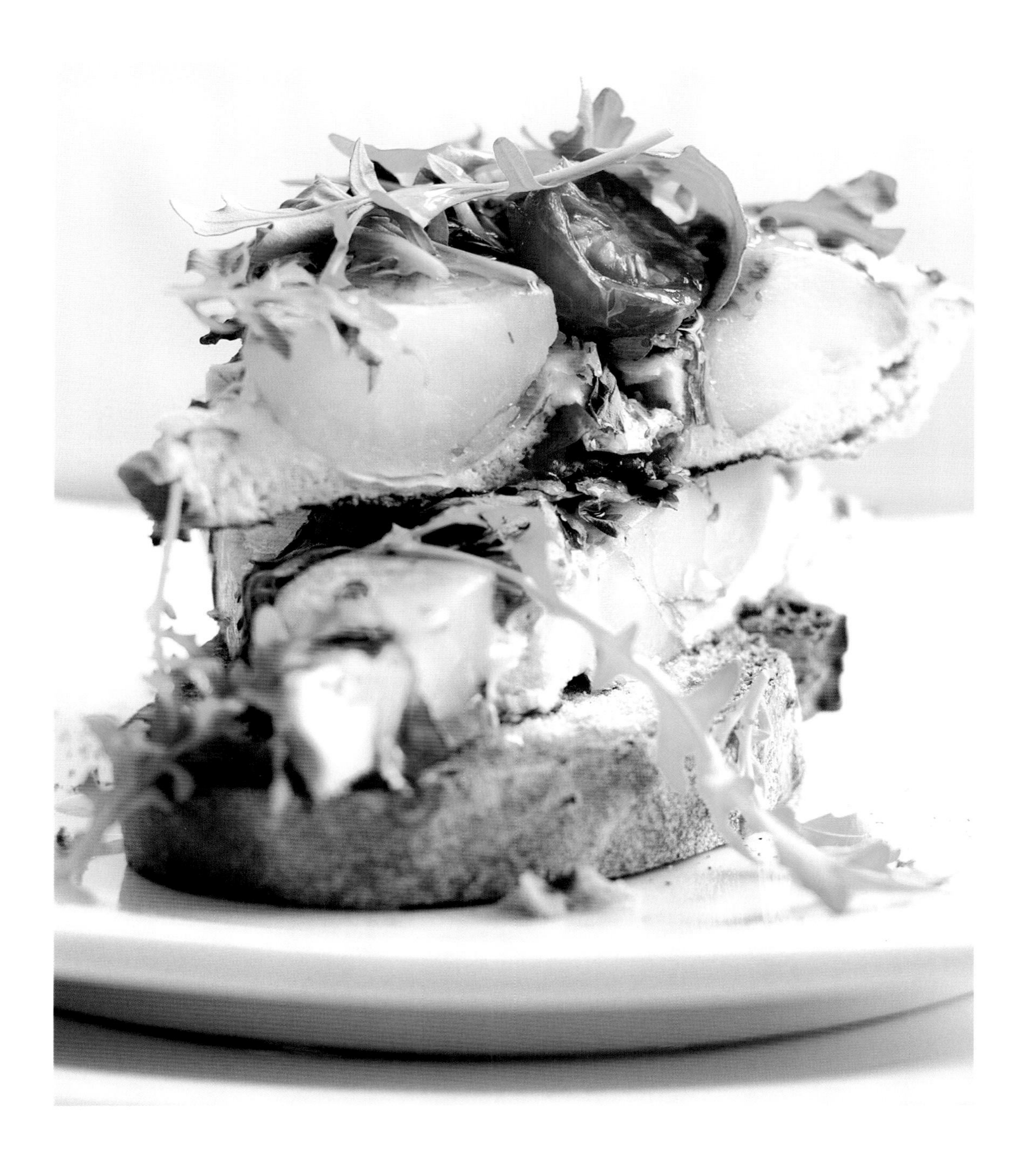

potato, rocket and tomato frittata

A frittata can be made quickly in the morning and you can basically add any ingredients you want, as long as the vegetables or meat are cooked before the egg is added to the pan. Once you're confident with the technique, why not experiment a little?

450 g (1 lb) baby new potatoes
1 tablespoon olive oil
1 garlic clove, crushed
50 g (2 oz) bag of wild rocket
175 g (6 oz) cherry tomatoes, halved
6 eggs, beaten
salt and freshly ground black pepper

Preparation: 20 minutes
Cooking time: 20–25 minutes
Serves 4

> Cut the potatoes in half or into chunks if necessary, then cook in a pan of lightly salted boiling water for 8–10 minutes. Drain.

> Heat the oil in a 20 cm (8 in) non-stick frying pan and fry the garlic over a low heat for 1 minute. Scatter over the potatoes, half the rocket and the cherry tomatoes. Pour over the eggs, season well with salt and freshly ground black pepper and cook over a medium heat for 3–4 minutes, until almost set. Use a wooden spatula to lift the frittata so that any unset egg can reach the base of the hot pan. When just set on the bottom, place under a preheated hot grill for 2–3 minutes to set the top. Scatter over the remaining rocket and serve immediately, with toasted crusty bread, if liked.

nutritional information calories 249 • fat 13 g • saturated fat 3.1 g • added sugar none • fibre 1.8 g • protein 14.1 g • salt 0.62 g • carbohydrate 20 g

healthy eating

> It may seem like a luxury to start the day with a substantial dish like this one, but it's actually a great way to get going in the morning. Rocket contains iron, folate, calcium, and vitamins C, beta-carotene and K; potatoes provide vitamin C, potassium and carbohydrate; and tomatoes contain anti-oxidants, including lycopene, beta-carotene and vitamin C.

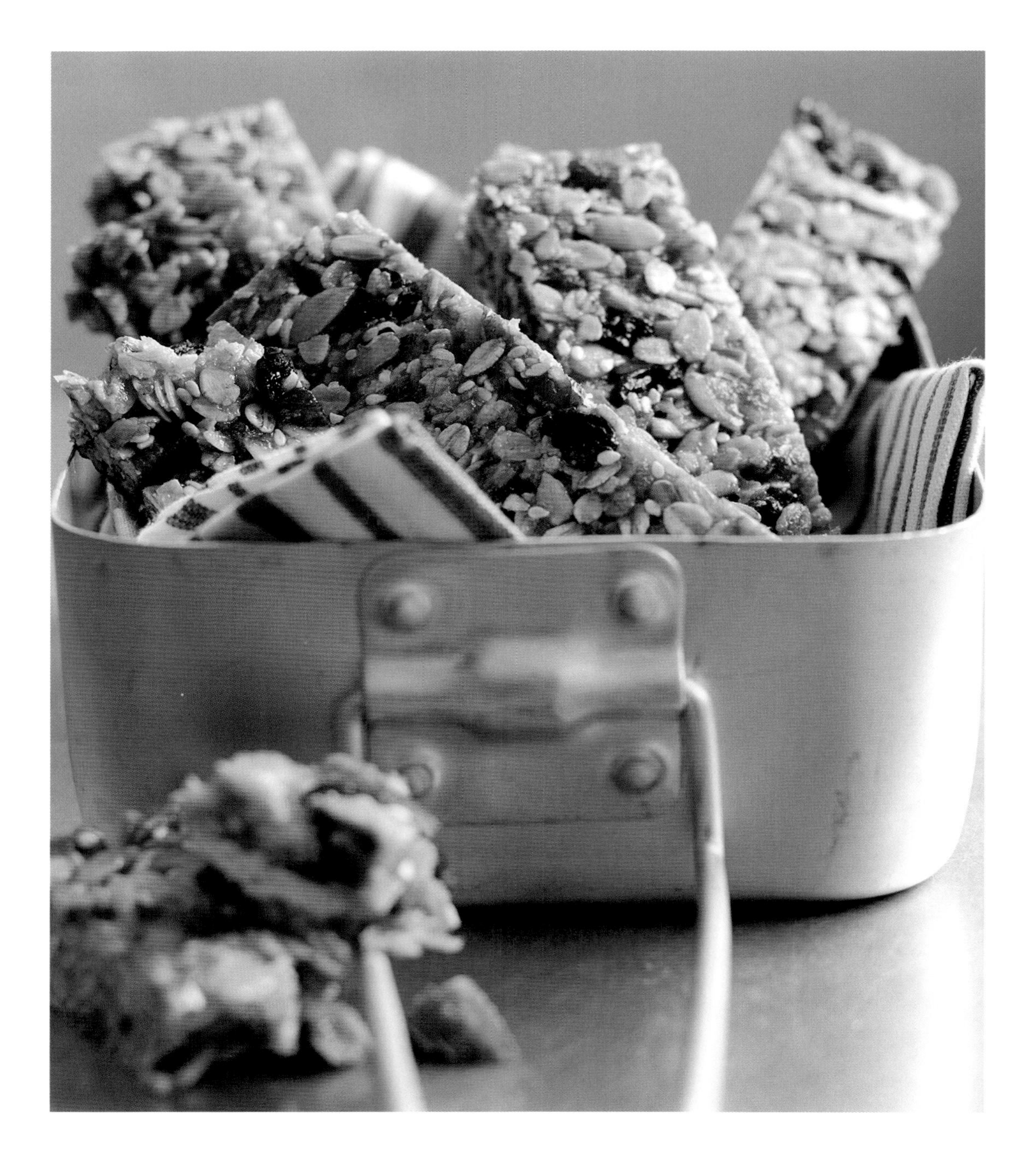

energy bars

These are called energy bars because energy is exactly what they will give you – powered by vitamins, minerals, such as zinc and iron, essential fatty acids, fibre and carbohydrates. They are also very tasty and a great favourite with the kids, too.

125 g (4 oz) dried apricots, roughly chopped
150 ml (¼ pint) orange juice
50 g (2 oz) butter
75 g (3 oz) runny honey
150 g (5 oz) demerara sugar
175 g (6 oz) porridge oats
50 g (2 oz) sultanas
75 g (3 oz) pecan nuts
50 g (2 oz) mixed pumpkin and sunflower seeds
25 g (1 oz) sesame seeds

Preparation: 20 minutes
Cooking time: 40 minutes
Makes 14 squares

- Preheat the oven to 190°C/375°F/Gas Mark 5. Line the base and sides of a 13 x 25 cm (5 x 10 in) cake tin with baking parchment.

- Put the apricots and orange juice in a large saucepan, bring to the boil and simmer gently, uncovered, for 20 minutes or until the apricots have softened. Transfer to a food processor and process to a thick smooth purée.

- Spoon the purée back into the pan and add the butter, honey and sugar. Cook over a low heat, stirring occasionally, for 5 minutes or until the sugar has dissolved.

- Stir in the remaining ingredients. Spoon into the prepared tin and bake for 15 minutes.

- When cool, remove from the tin and discard the lining paper. Cut into 14 squares.

nutritional information calories 230 • fat 10.3 g • saturated fat 2.5 g • added sugar 15.3 g • fibre 2.7 g • protein 4.4 g • salt 0.09 g • carbohydrate 32 g

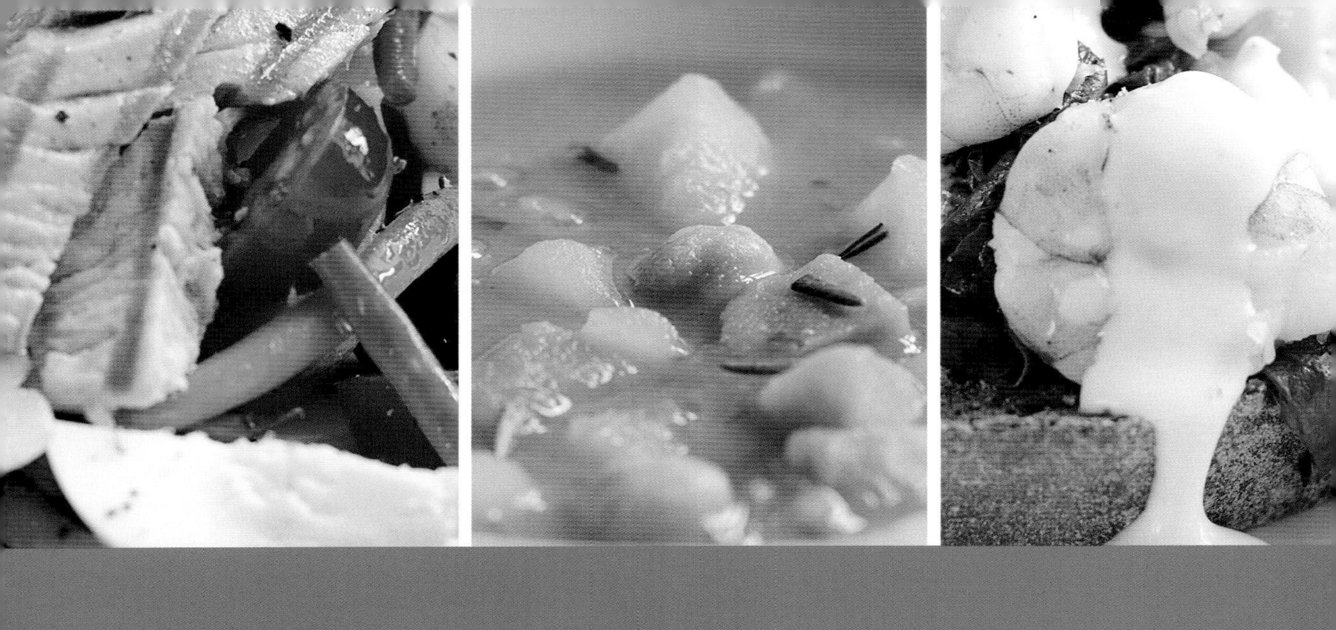

light bites

To most of us lunch consists of a sandwich and perhaps some crisps, snatched on the run while we're at work or looking after the kids. For athletes too, lunch is often a quick snack between training sessions, so it needs to be easy to eat yet packed full of nutrients and energy. This chapter is full of delicious ideas to inspire you. With just a little time spent planning you'll find your lunch menu can be expanded to include tasty salads, wraps and even hot sandwiches ... delicious!

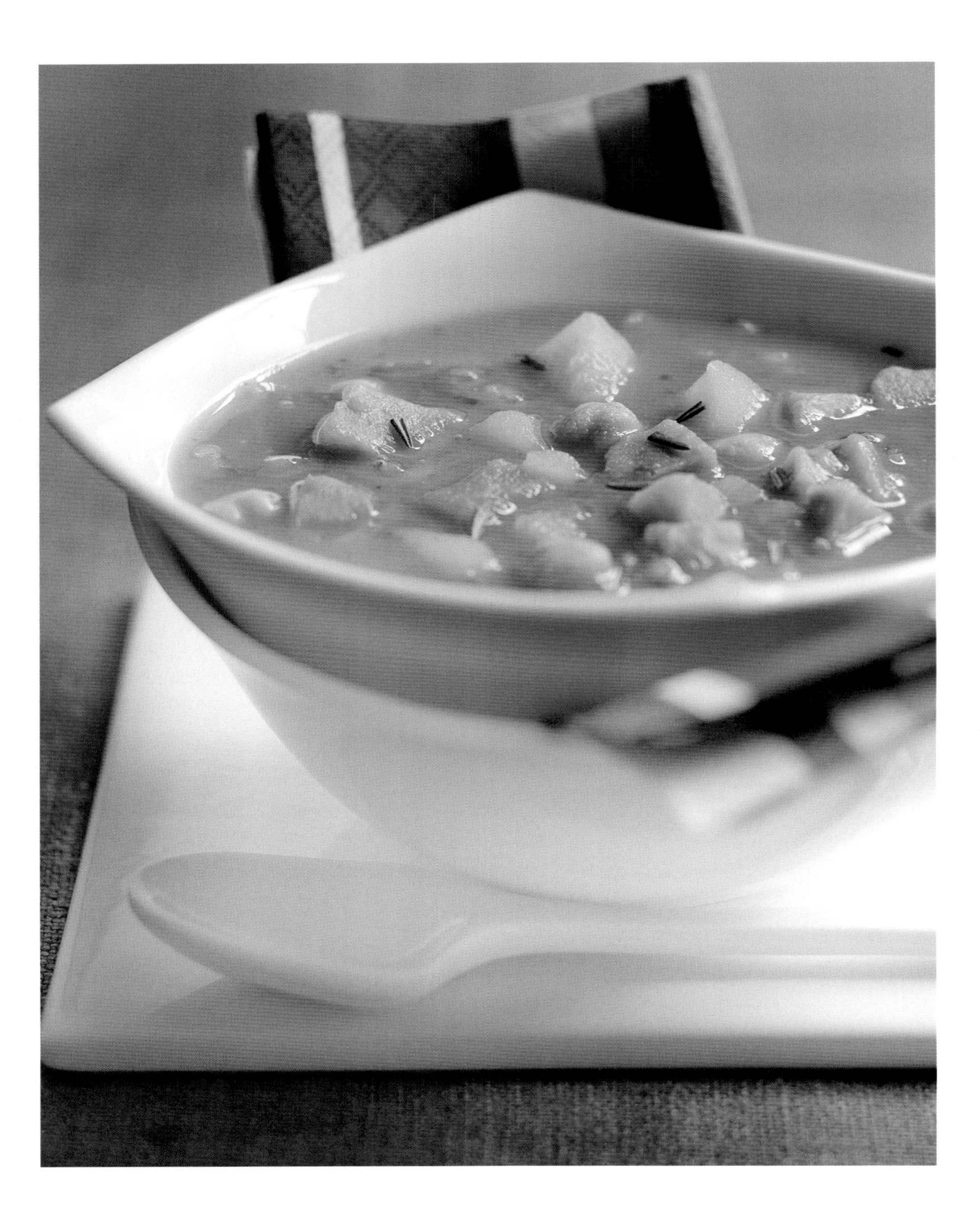

sweet potato and chick-pea soup

Choose the brown-skinned, pink-fleshed variety of sweet potatoes as they are far better for you than the red-skinned, white-fleshed variety. They are a great energy-booster vegetable, full of goodness, with high levels of beta-carotene, which enhances the immune system and deals with viral infections.

1 tablespoon olive oil
1 large onion, finely chopped
1 large baking potato, peeled and finely diced
1 large brown-skinned, pink-fleshed sweet potato, about 350 g (12 oz), peeled and finely diced
1 garlic clove, crushed
1 fresh rosemary sprig, leaves removed and finely chopped
850 ml (1½ pints) vegetable stock
410 g can of chick-peas, drained and rinsed
salt and freshly ground black pepper

Preparation: 20 minutes
Cooking time: 30 minutes
Serves 4

> Heat the oil in a large frying pan and fry the onion, potato and sweet potato for 4–5 minutes, until the onion is just beginning to soften. Stir in the garlic and rosemary and cook for 1 minute.

> Pour over the stock, bring to the boil, cover and simmer for 15 minutes.

> Use a potato masher to mash some of the soup or blend with a hand blender until nearly smooth but with some texture.

> Stir in the chick-peas and simmer for a further 5 minutes. Season to taste and serve with crusty bread.

nutritional information calories 238 • fat 5.1 g • saturated fat 0.5 g • added sugar none • fibre 6 g • protein 8.3 g • salt 1.39 g • carbohydrate 42 g

healthy eating

> Sweet potatoes are an excellent source of beta-carotene and carbohydrate. They also contain good quantities of potassium and vitamin C.

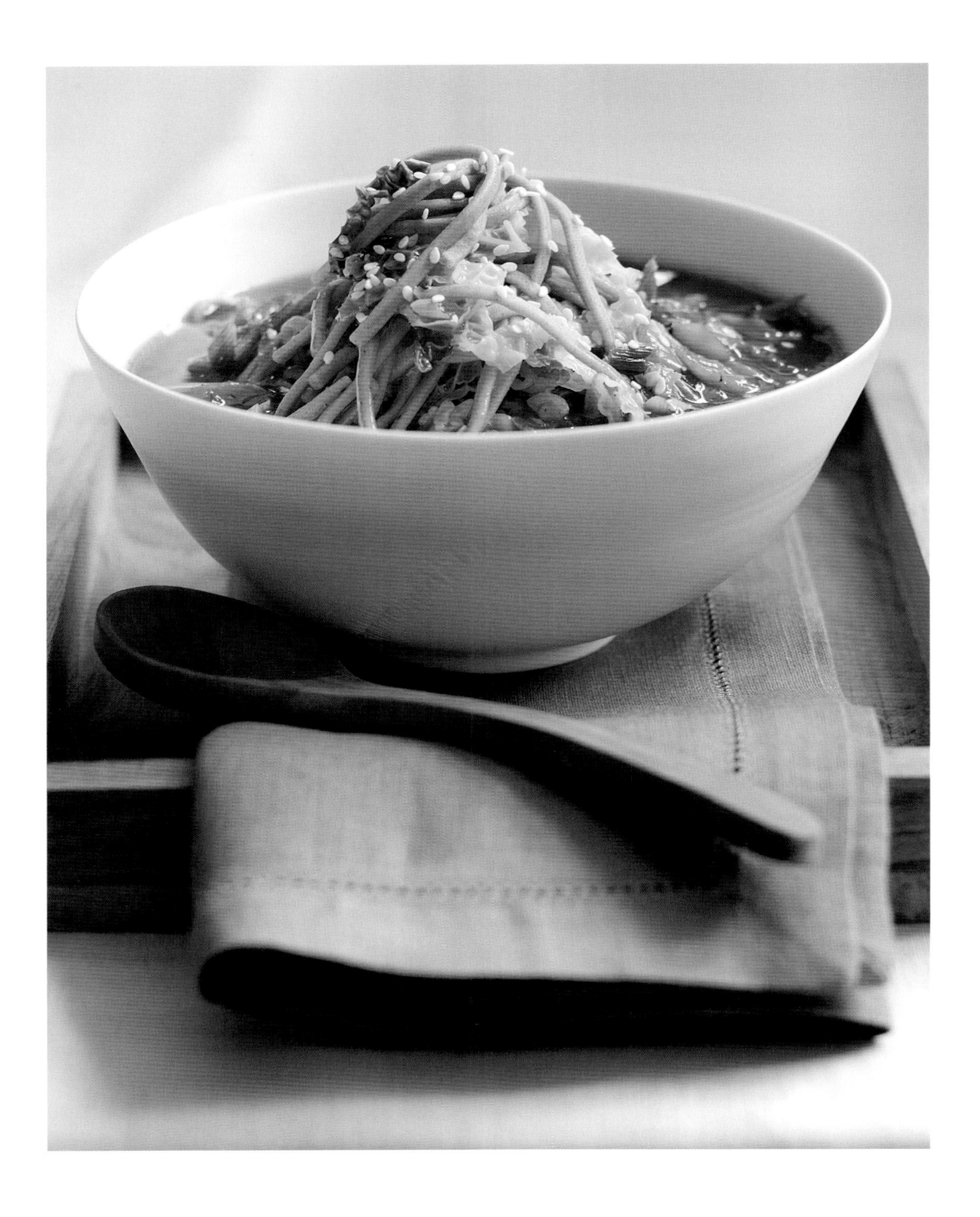

soba noodle broth with spring greens

Boost your immune system, give yourself an energy boost and soothe away stress with this action-packed soup. Soba noodles provide the carbohydrate, garlic protects the immune system and both garlic and ginger may help clear the nasal passages – a clear winner with a little bit of everything.

175 g (6 oz) soba noodles
250 g (9 oz) spring greens or savoy cabbage, finely shredded
1 tablespoon vegetable oil
1 bunch of spring onions, trimmed and sliced
2 garlic cloves, crushed
1 teaspoon minced chillies
2 teaspoons minced ginger
2 teaspoons soy sauce
160 g sachet of black bean stir-fry sauce
900 ml (1½ pints) hot vegetable stock
2 teaspoons sesame seeds, toasted

Preparation: 15 minutes
Cooking time: 16–20 minutes
Serves 4

> Cook the noodles in plenty of lightly salted boiling water for 5 minutes until just tender. Add the shredded greens and cook for a further 1 minute. Drain, return to the pan and cover with a lid.

> Heat the oil in a large saucepan and fry the spring onions for 1–2 minutes, stirring occasionally. Add the garlic, chillies, ginger, soy sauce, black bean sauce and stock and bring to the boil. Then simmer for 5 minutes.

> Twist the noodles and spring greens around a large carving fork and pile into individual serving bowls. Spoon over the black bean mixture and serve scattered with sesame seeds.

nutritional information calories 281 • fat 8.3 g • saturated fat 1.2 g • added sugar 1.9 g • fibre 4.8 g • protein 12.1 g • salt 3.78 g • carbohydrate 42.1 g

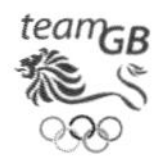

Sharron Davies's

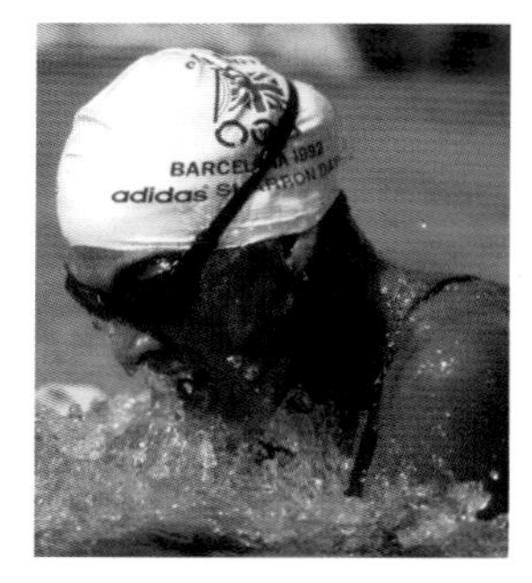

chicken caesar salad

I love caesar salad – it always reminds me of holidays sitting in the sun. I often buy a reduced-fat caesar dressing if I'm feeling lazy: it's always handy to have in the fridge. You can, of course, grate over some Parmesan – a little goes a long way!

2 thick slices of granary bread, crusts removed, crumb cut into cubes
1 teaspoon cajun seasoning
2 tablespoons olive oil
1 garlic clove, crushed
1 large cos lettuce
4 tablespoons half-fat crème fraîche
1 tablespoon lemon juice
2 teaspoons Worcestershire sauce
1 teaspoon Dijon mustard
2 large cooked skinless, boneless chicken breasts, thinly sliced
salt and freshly ground black pepper

Preparation: 15 minutes
Cooking time: 10 minutes
Serves 4

> Preheat the oven to 220°C/425°F/Gas Mark 7. Toss the bread cubes with the cajun seasoning, 1 tablespoon of the olive oil and the garlic. Spread on to a baking sheet and bake for 8 minutes, until golden and crisp.

> Trim the lettuce, then tear into pieces and toss with the spicy croûtons. Pile into four individual serving bowls. Mix together the remaining olive oil, crème fraîche, lemon juice, Worcestershire sauce and Dijon mustard and season to taste. Drizzle over the cos lettuce and arrange the chicken slices on top to serve.

nutritional information calories 247 • fat 12 g • saturated fat 3 g • added sugar none • fibre 2 g • protein 24 g • salt 1.18 g • carbohydrate 12 g

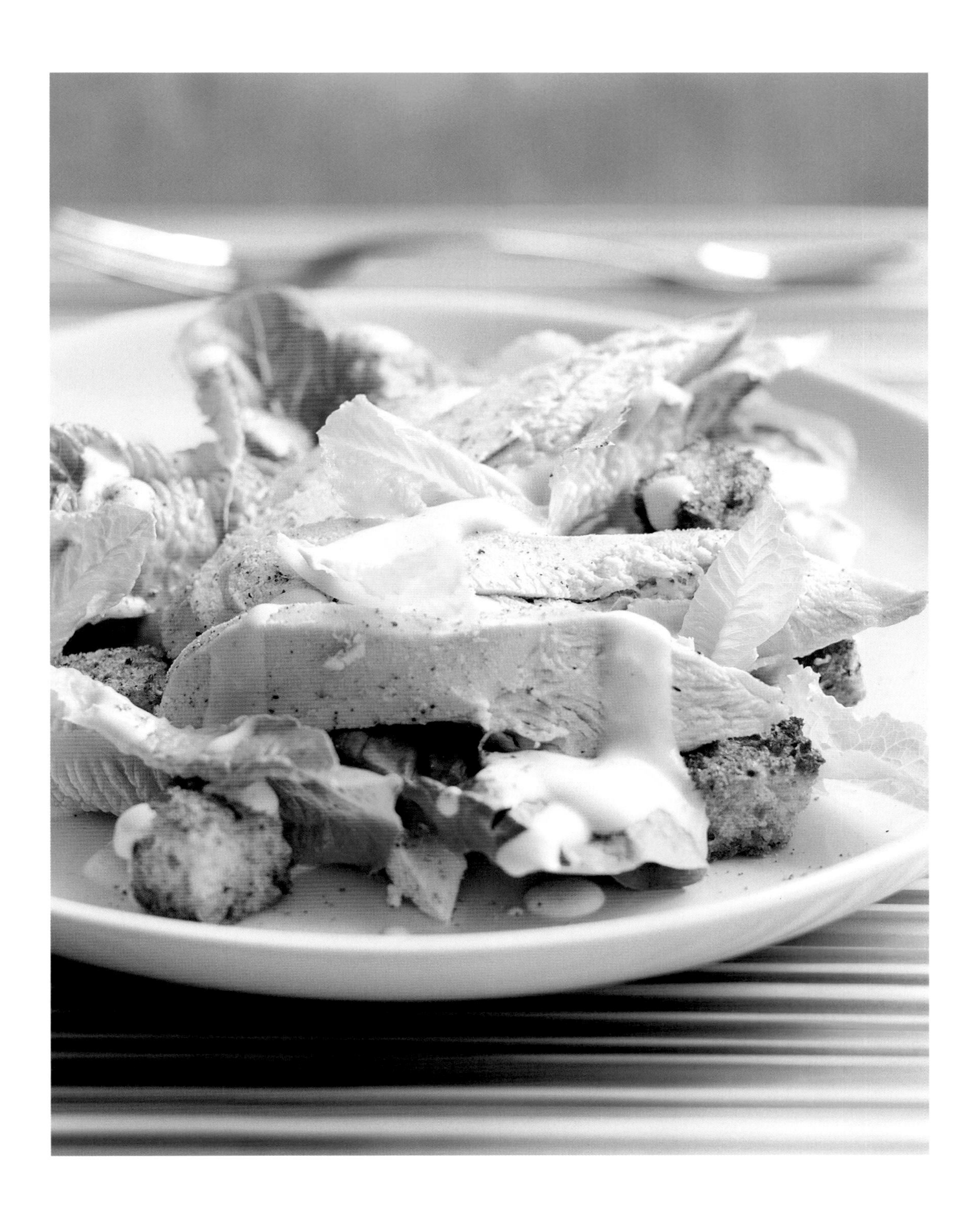

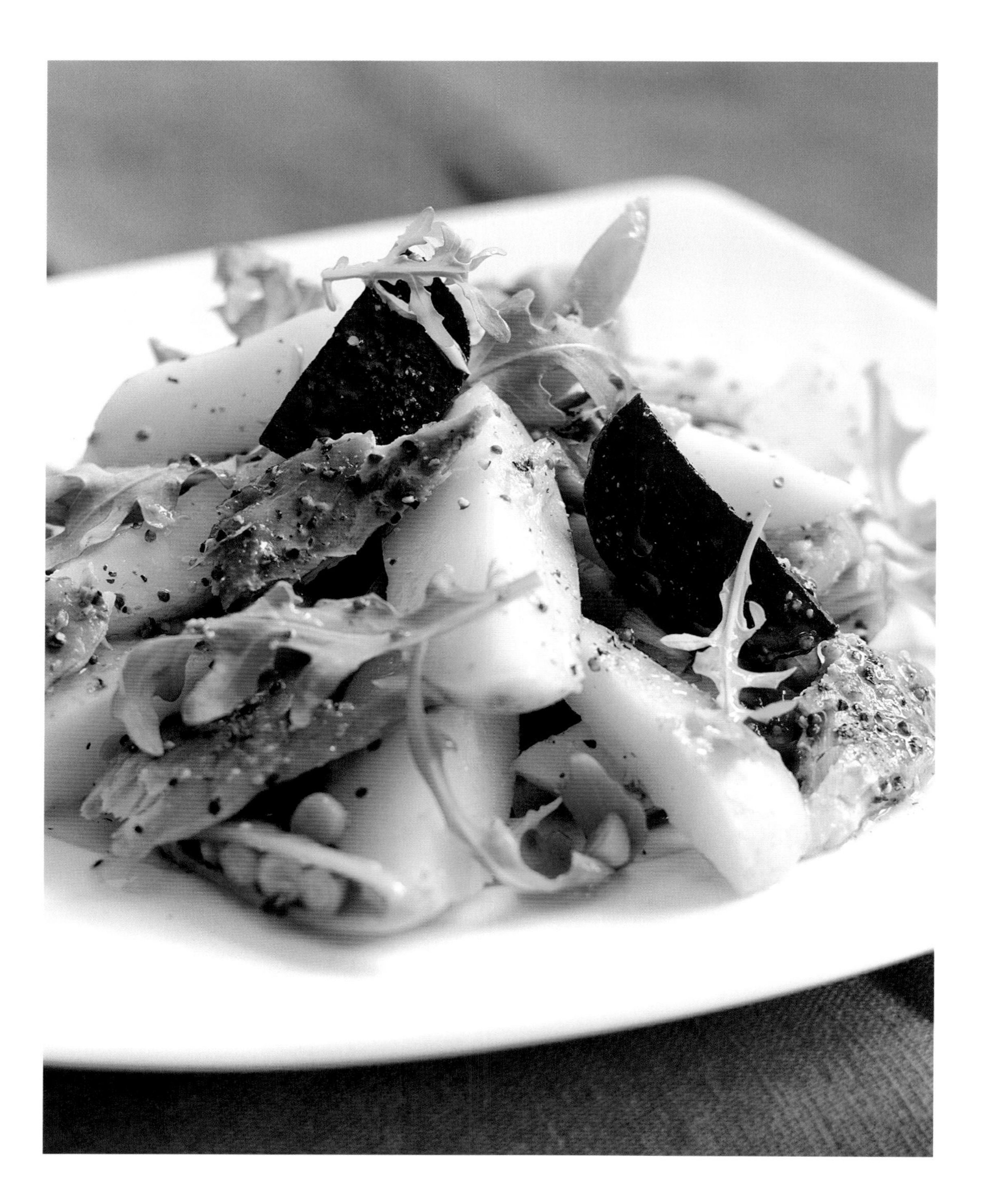

new potato, smoked mackerel and beetroot salad

We all know that oily fish is good for us, containing as it does essential omega-3 fatty acids and vitamins A and D. This delicious salad would make a wonderful starter for six people. Ring the changes with smoked trout or oak-smoked salmon.

2 tablespoons olive oil
1 tablespoon red wine vinegar
½ teaspoon caster sugar
1 heaped teaspoon wholegrain mustard
450 g (1 lb) new potatoes, quartered lengthways
125 g (4 oz) sugarsnap peas, shredded lengthways
50 g bag of wild rocket
2 cooked fresh beetroot dipped in malt vinegar, cut into wedges
250 g (9 oz) peppered smoked mackerel, flaked
salt and freshly ground black pepper

Preparation: 15 minutes
Cooking time: 8–10 minutes
Serves 4

> Mix together the olive oil, red wine vinegar, sugar and wholegrain mustard and season to taste with salt and freshly ground black pepper. Chill until ready to use.

> Cook the potatoes in a pan of lightly salted boiling water for 8–10 minutes until just tender. Drain and run under cold water, drain again and then toss with the dressing. Stir in the sugarsnap peas and spoon on to a serving dish.

> Scatter over the rocket and beetroot. Flake over the peppered mackerel and serve warm or cold.

nutritional information calories 377 • fat 25.6 g • saturated fat 5.5 g • added sugar 0.7 g • fibre 2.2 g • protein 15.7 g • salt 1.68 g • carbohydrate 22 g

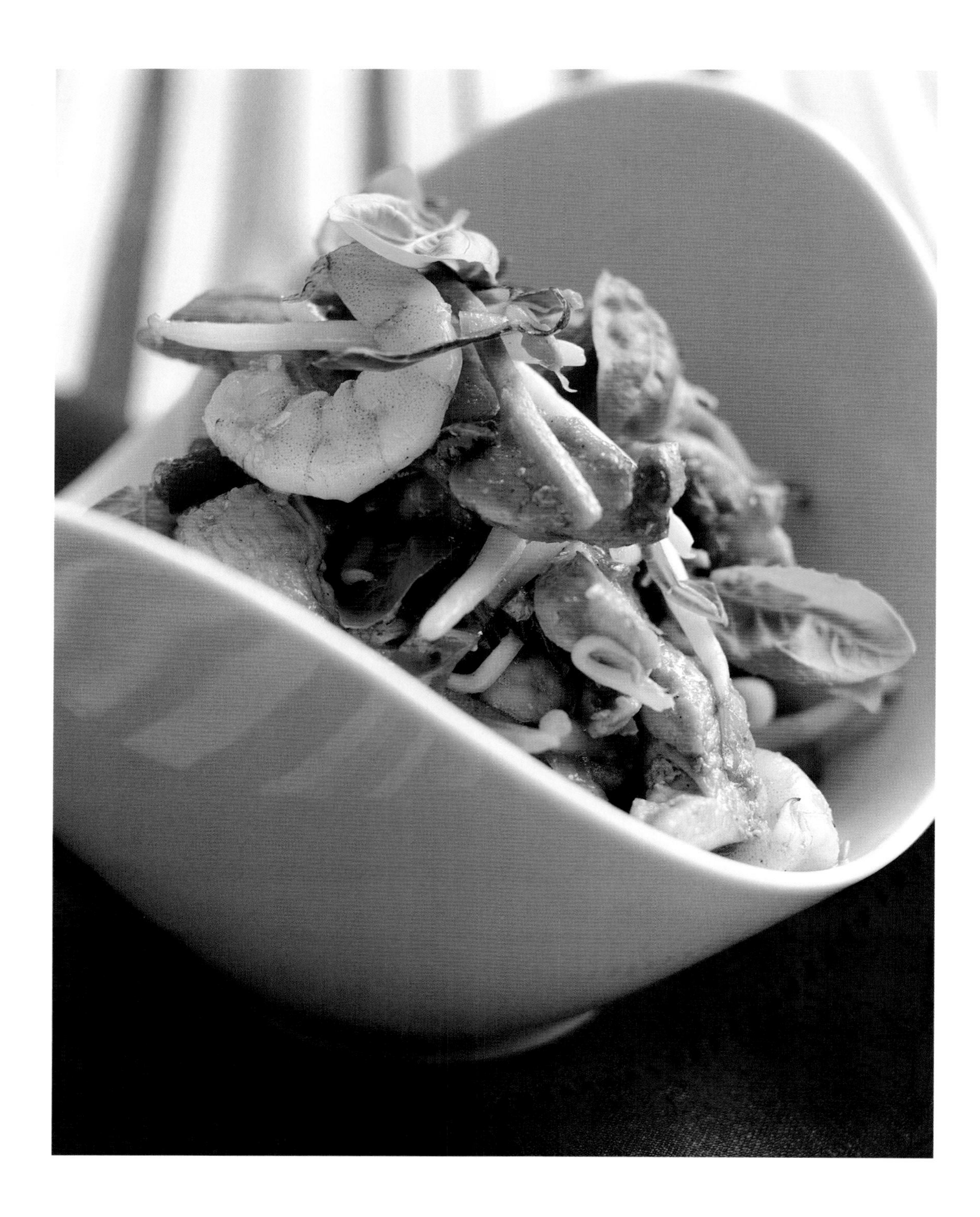

hot 'n' spicy thai chicken and prawn salad

Hot and spicy and cool and crunchy – this salad has everything. It's hard to believe that it only takes minutes to cook. To make it go further and for extra carbohydrate I often add a handful of soaked rice vermicelli noodles.

1 tablespoon groundnut oil
450 g (1 lb) skinless, boneless chicken breasts, cut into thin strips
1 small onion, very finely chopped
4 garlic cloves, crushed
2 tablespoons Thai fish sauce
2 teaspoons soy sauce
2 teaspoons caster sugar
2–3 red Thai chillies, seeded and very thinly shredded
125 g (4 oz) shelled, cooked jumbo prawns
fresh lime juice, to taste
200 g bag of shredded vegetable salad or beansprout stir-fry mix
handful of basil leaves, to garnish

Preparation: 20 minutes
Cooking time: 15 minutes
Serves 4

> Heat the oil in a wok or large frying pan until hot and smoking. Stir-fry the chicken for 5 minutes. Drain the chicken, saving the juices.

> Add the onion and garlic to the pan and stir-fry for 2 minutes. Add the chicken juices (if you haven't got a lot of chicken juices, add 1 tablespoon cold water) and stir-fry for a further minute.

> Return the chicken to the pan, with the fish sauce, soy sauce, sugar and chillies and stir-fry for 5 minutes, until the chicken is browned and the sauce reduced to a sticky glaze. Stir in the prawns, and lime juice to taste, and stir to coat. Toss in the shredded salad or beansprout stir-fry mix, garnish with basil leaves and serve.

nutritional information calories 212 • fat 4.6 g • saturated fat 1 g • added sugar 2.8 g • fibre 1 g • protein 36.1 g • salt 3.25 g • carbohydrate 7 g

“I required a 6000-calorie diet and that’s a huge amount of food.” > **Steve Redgrave**

car

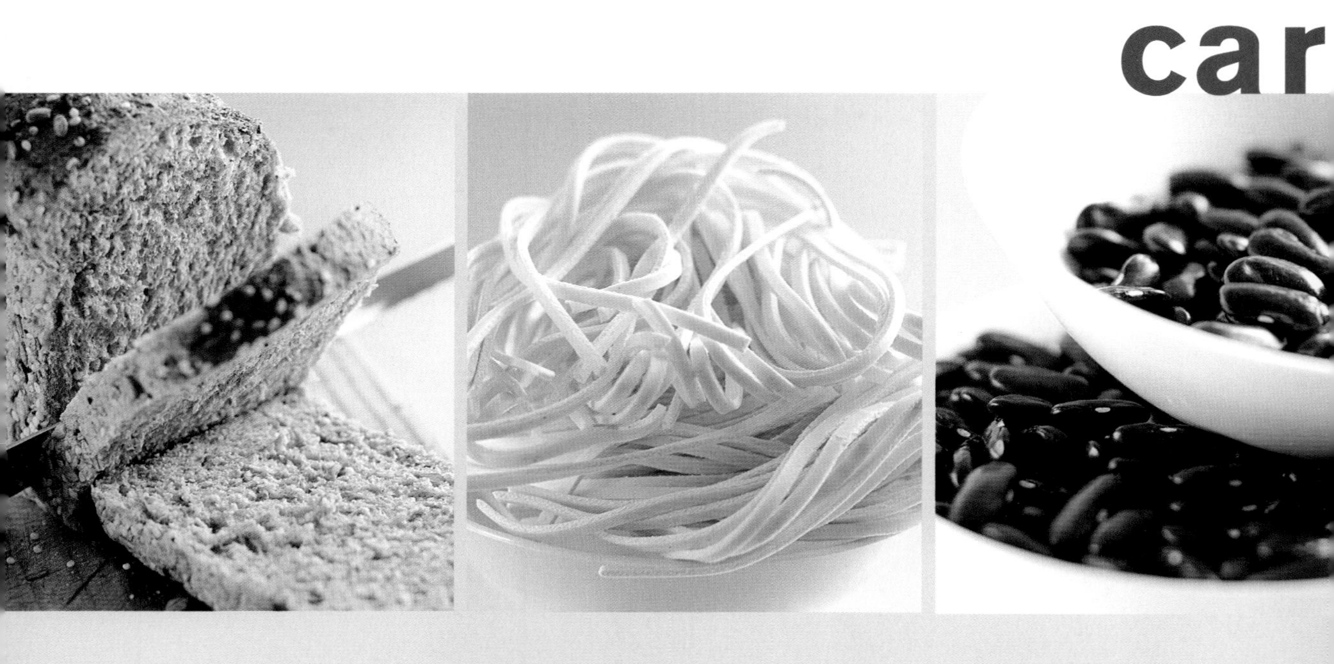

“It was vital that I maintained my energy levels for training and racing.” > **Steve Redgrave**

Five-times Olympic gold medallist rower Sir Steve Redgrave CBE had to be full of energy and ready to power his way to the finishing line when racing. In order to prepare himself it was vital that Steve ate plenty of the right kind of foods so that he had a bank of stored energy for the hours of exhaustive daily training. The fuel for his training came from starchy carbohydrate that can be found in a

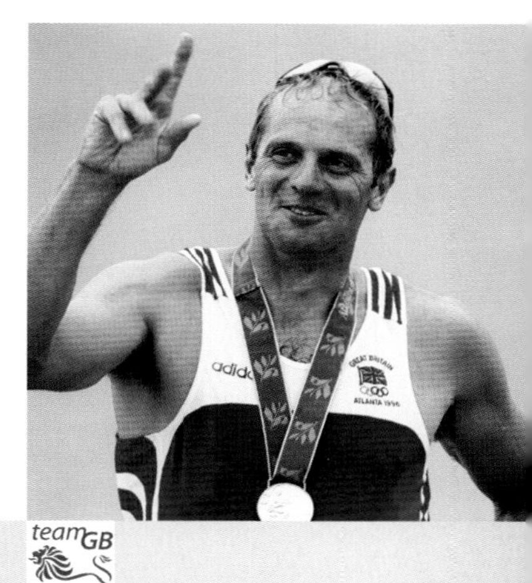

bohydrates

number of foods, especially pasta, potatoes, rice, bread, and breakfast cereal. Despite eating large amounts of these foods, athletes like Steve still need to include some sugary carbohydrates to fuel their muscles' need for energy. Sugars are less bulky then starches and so achieving a high-carbohydrate diet becomes easier. A look at Steve's food diary (see right) shows that if he did not add sugar to his porridge he would have needed to eat another two Weetabix!

The amount of carbohydrate you need daily depends on how active you are. For example, a growing teenager may need eleven or more portions a day, whereas a sedentary woman would need only five or six. Athletes with high energy needs may need fourteen or more portions every day. Foods rich in starchy or unrefined carbohydrate are vital sources of energy for us all and should make up the largest portions of a balanced diet. By choosing wholemeal bread, brown rice and wholegrain cereals we can ensure not only a good intake of carbohydrate but also B vitamins, fibre and minerals such as magnesium and zinc. The list below should give you an idea of what is meant by a portion of carbohydrate. Each entry is a single portion:

- 1 slice of bread
- 1 egg-sized potato
- 2 tablespoons pasta or rice
- 3 tablespoons breakfast cereal

Steve's food diary

> **Breakfast**

A large jug of juice and four Weetabix, followed by a bowl of porridge with a lot of brown sugar between training sessions.

> **Lunch**

A large pasta dish and a pudding with another jug of juice.

> **Main meal**

Spaghetti bolognese followed by rice pudding or apple pie and ice-cream, and more cereal before going to bed.

> **In between**

I'd pick up some chocolate or doughnuts. Alcohol was generally ruled out, although if I was at a dinner I might have a glass of champagne or wine.

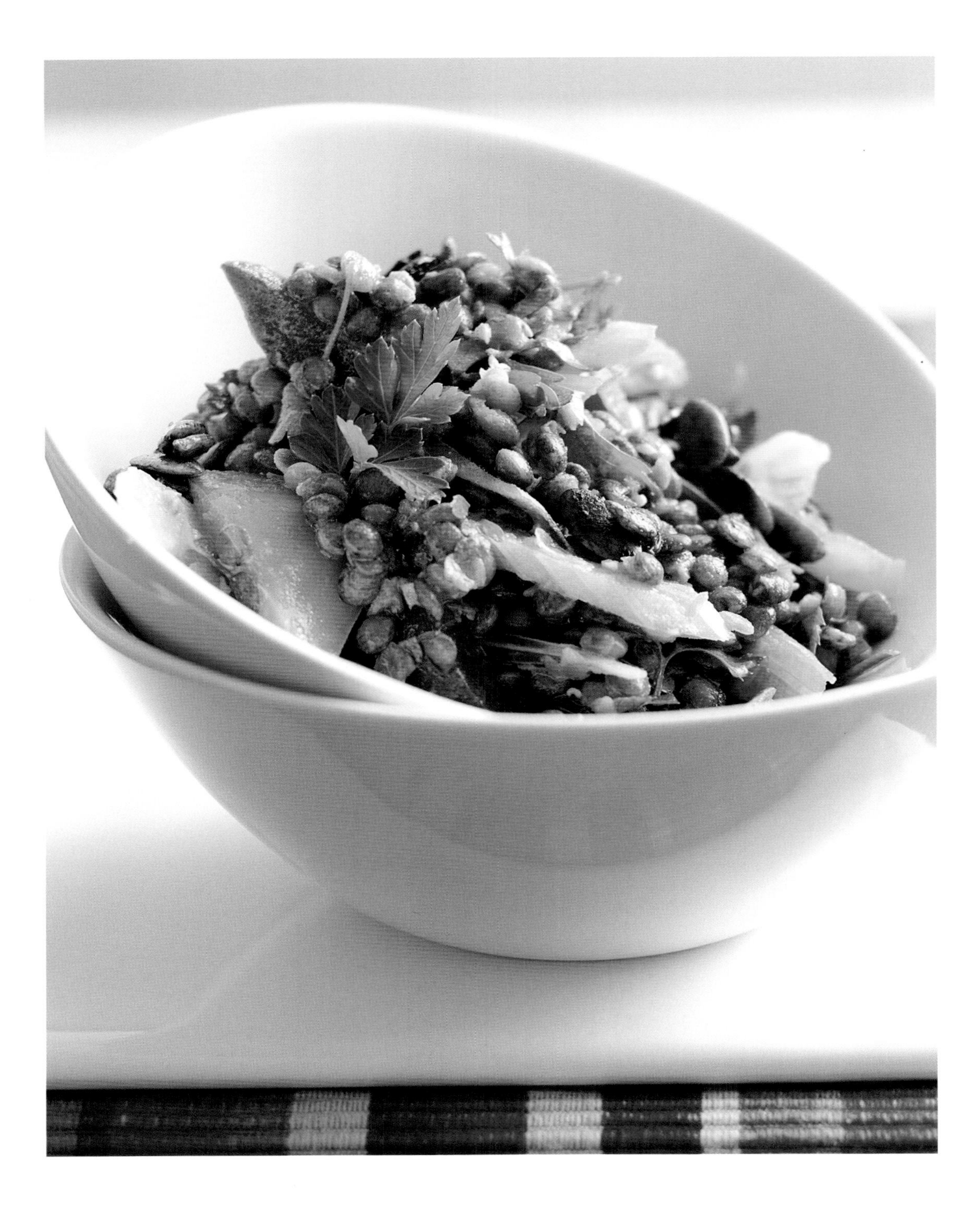

crunchy puy lentil salad

Lentils are an underestimated ingredient – a good source of zinc, iron, fibre, protein and slow-release carbohydrate. These Puy lentils soak up the dressing to create a tasty salad that could be served warm with grilled meat, or cold with goats' cheese on crusty bread.

125 g (4 oz) mixed seeds, such as sunflower, pumpkin and sesame
1 tablespoon soy sauce
1 tablespoon runny honey
250 g (9 oz) Puy lentils
2 tablespoons extra virgin olive oil
1 tablespoon lemon juice
2 teaspoons Dijon mustard
2 garlic cloves, crushed
1 large red onion, cut into thin wedges
1 large red pepper, seeded and cut into small chunks
1 large yellow pepper, seeded and cut into small chunks
4 celery sticks, trimmed and sliced diagonally
large handful of torn flatleaf parsley
salt and freshly ground black pepper

Preparation: 25 minutes
Cooking time: 20–25 minutes
Serves 4

> In a dry frying pan, toast the mixed seeds for 2–3 minutes, stirring continuously until lightly browned. Pour over the soy sauce and runny honey and quickly give it a stir (the seeds will stick together to begin with but, as the mixture heats and dries, they will separate). Leave to cool and then break up into small pieces.

> Place the lentils in a saucepan and cover with cold water, bring to the boil and boil rapidly for 5 minutes. Reduce the heat and cook for 20 minutes, until the lentils are tender.

> Drain the lentils and return to the pan. Stir in the olive oil, lemon juice, Dijon mustard and garlic, stir well and leave to cool (the lentils will absorb some of the dressing).

> When cold, stir in the remaining ingredients, including the toasted seeds. Season to taste.

nutritional information calories 446 • fat 20 g • saturated fat 2.7 g • added sugar 2.9 g • fibre 9.9 g • protein 22.7 g • salt 1.22 g • carbohydrate 47 g

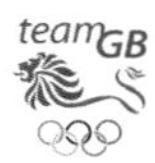

Audley Harrison's

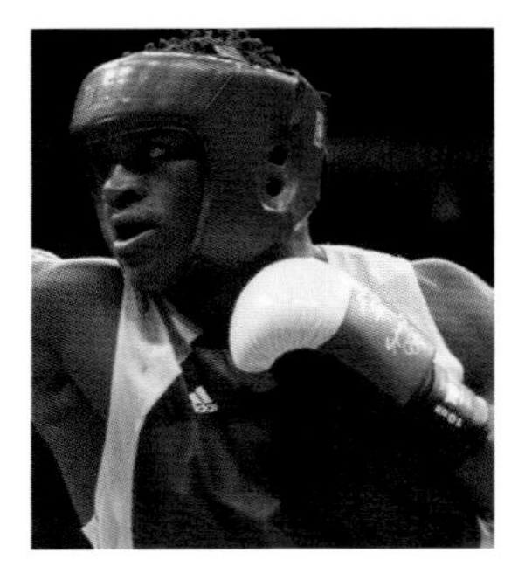

steak sandwich with mustard sauce

Famously winning Olympic gold on a cooked breakfast, Audley clearly likes meat. This snack packs a punch being low in fat, high in carbohydrate, and the steak is a great source of iron-rich protein. It is sure to be a hit with friends as Sunday brunch.

125 g (4 oz) quark (semi-skimmed-milk soft cheese)
4 tablespoons skimmed milk
2 tablespoons wholegrain mustard
25 g (1 oz) gherkins, chopped
small handful of chopped parsley
2 onions, thinly sliced
1 tablespoon soft dark brown sugar
2 garlic cloves, crushed
4 ciabatta rolls, split
1 teaspoon olive oil
4 thin pieces of flash-fry steak, about 250 g (9 oz) in total
salt and freshly ground black pepper
shredded iceberg lettuce and sliced tomatoes, to serve

Preparation: 20 minutes
Cooking time: 20–25 minutes
Serves 4

> Beat the quark with the milk until smooth and creamy. Stir in the mustard, gherkins and parsley and season to taste with salt and freshly ground black pepper.

> Place the onions, sugar and garlic in a frying pan and add just enough water to cover. Bring to the boil and simmer gently for about 10–12 minutes, stirring occasionally, until golden brown and sticky.

> Heat a griddle pan until smoking. Toast the ciabatta on the griddle and then set aside.

> Brush the olive oil over both sides of the steak and season well with freshly ground black pepper. Sear on the griddle for 2 minutes on one side, turn over and cook for a further minute.

> Pile the lettuce, tomato and steak on to the bottom halves of the ciabatta, spoon over the onions and mustard sauce and serve topped with the other halves of ciabatta.

nutritional information calories 289 • fat 6.5 g • saturated fat 1.5 g • added sugar 3.8 g • fibre 2.6 g • protein 25.3 g • salt 1.48 g • carbohydrate 34 g

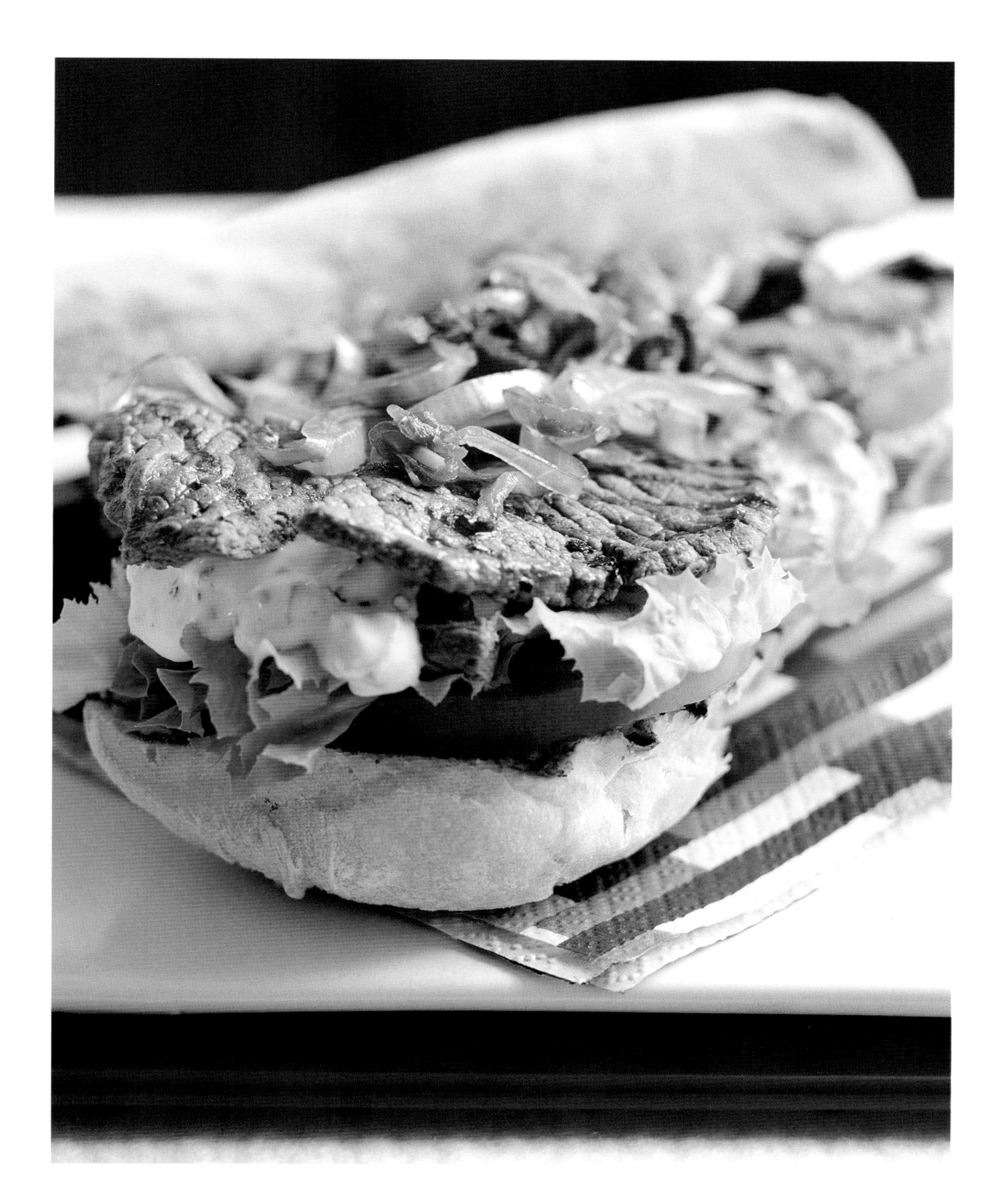

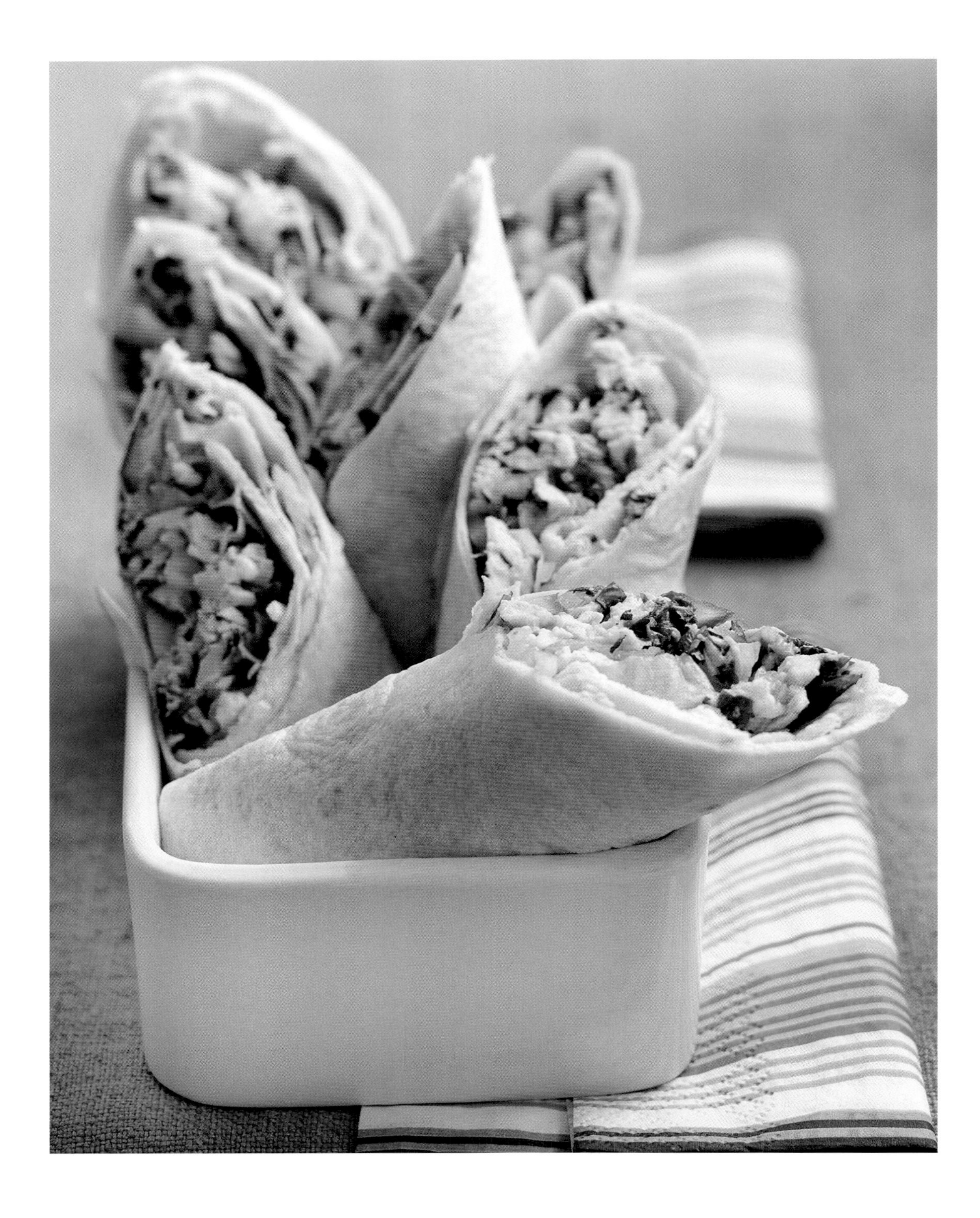

chicken salad wraps

The great thing about these wraps is that they make a little chicken go a long way. Moist, crisp, sweet, cool and tasty all in one mouthful – a delicious fusion of different flavours and one of my favourite sandwiches.

½ cucumber
2 cooked skinless, boneless chicken breasts, shredded
large handful of fresh coriander leaves
small handful of fresh mint leaves
1 tablespoon Thai fish sauce
1 teaspoon sesame oil
juice and finely grated zest of 2 limes
¼ small iceberg lettuce, finely shredded
6 tablespoons plum sauce
6 x 20 cm (8 in) flour tortillas
salt and freshly ground black pepper

Preparation: 15 minutes
Cooking time: none
Makes 6

> Halve the cucumber lengthways and, using a teaspoon, scoop out the seeds. Then cut into long thin batons.

> Toss the shredded chicken with the coriander, mint, fish sauce, sesame oil, lime zest and juice and iceberg lettuce. Season to taste with salt and pepper.

> Spread 1 tablespoon of the plum sauce over each of the tortillas. Spoon the chicken mixture on top, scatter over some cucumber and roll up. Halve and serve with juice and fresh fruit.

nutritional information calories 270 • fat 5.9 g • saturated fat 1 g • added sugar 8.4 g • fibre 1.8 g • protein 16.6 g • salt 2.84 g • carbohydrate 40 g

healthy eating

> Chicken contains all of the B vitamins which are so important for sport performance and good health.

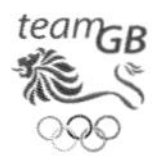

Georgina Harland's niçoise salad

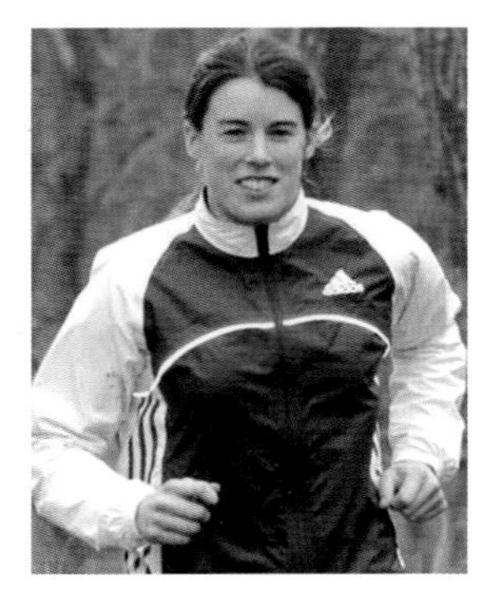

The main advantage of this meal is it can be served hot or cold and can be prepared in advance. It is also easy to take with me, which is so important in my sport since I am on the go from morning until night, with little time to prepare a decent meal.

1 medium egg
4 baby new potatoes, halved lengthways
125 g (4 oz) fine green beans, trimmed
4 cherry tomatoes, halved
5 pitted black olives
small handful of torn flatleaf parsley
1 tablespoon extra virgin olive oil
1 fresh tuna steak, about 150 g (5 oz)
salt and freshly ground black pepper

Preparation: 15–20 minutes
Cooking time: 25–30 minutes
Serves 1

> Place the egg in a small pan of cold water, bring to the boil and simmer for 7–9 minutes. Drain and refresh in plenty of cold water.

> Cook the new potatoes in a pan of lightly salted boiling water for 7 minutes. Add the green beans and cook for a further 2 minutes or until the potatoes are just tender. Drain and toss in a mixing bowl with the cherry tomatoes, olives and parsley.

> Heat a griddle pan until hot and smoking. Brush some of the oil over both sides of the tuna steak and season with salt and freshly ground black pepper. Griddle for 2 minutes on each side.

> Meanwhile, shell the egg and cut into quarters. Toss the remaining olive oil with the potato mixture, season to taste and spoon onto a serving plate. Arrange the egg quarters over the top. Slice the tuna and arrange over the top of the salad. Serve with a warm crusty brown baguette.

nutritional information calories 482 • fat 25.9 g • saturated fat 5.6 g • added sugar none • fibre 4.1 g • protein 45.7 g • salt 1.5 g • carbohydrate 18 g

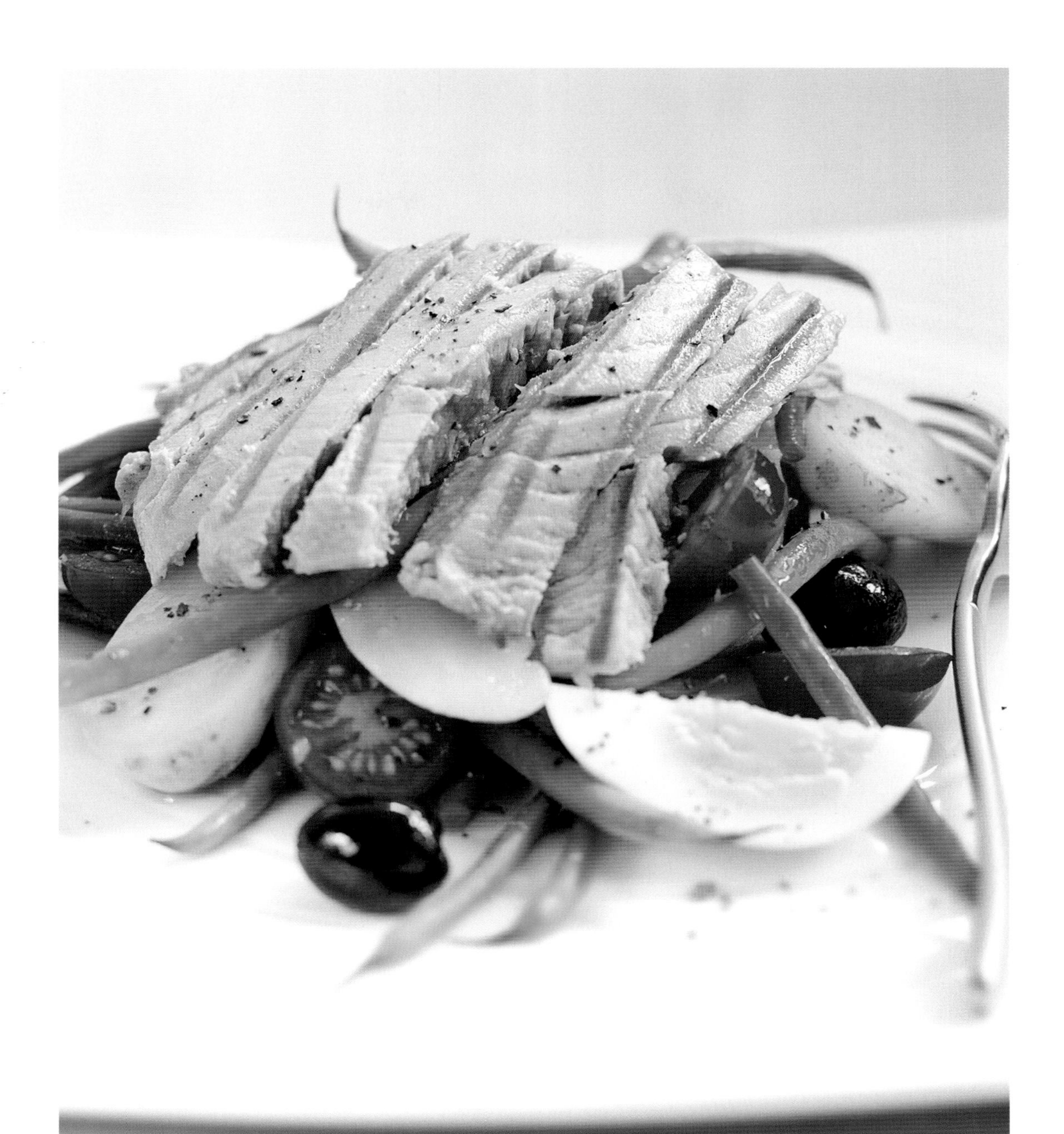

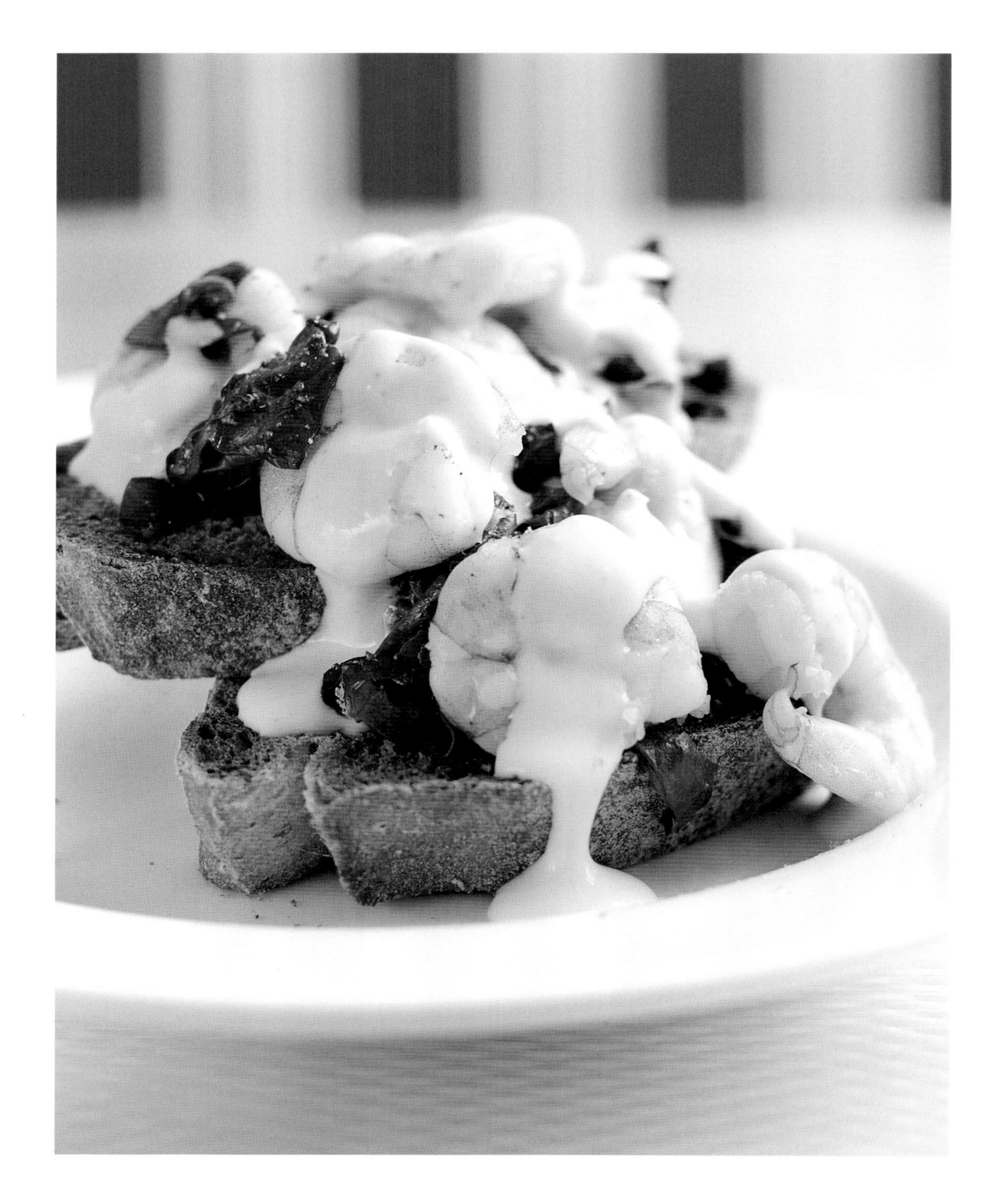

hot and creamy prawns on toast

Prawns are a real favourite of mine and I put them in everything, including on toast. This is a great combination for a quick, no-nonsense yet healthy supper. Bags of frozen prawns are a great stand-by food – I always make sure I've got one in the freezer.

4 thick slices of crusty wholemeal or granary bread
2 teaspoons olive oil
1 small red onion, cut into thin wedges
200 g (7 oz) shelled, raw jumbo tiger prawns, thawed if frozen
2 tablespoons half-fat crème fraîche
1 heaped teaspoon Dijon mustard
juice of ½ small lemon
125 g (4 oz) baby spinach leaves
lemon wedges, to serve (optional)

Preparation: 5 minutes
Cooking time: 10 minutes
Serves 2

> Toast the wholemeal or granary bread until golden on both sides and then wrap in a clean cloth to keep warm.

> Heat the oil in a wok or large frying pan and fry the onion for 2–3 minutes until beginning to soften. Tip in the prawns and stir-fry for 2 minutes, until pink. Add the crème fraîche, mustard and lemon juice and stir well to combine. Season to taste, then stir in the spinach leaves until just wilted.

> Arrange the toast on two serving plates and spoon over the hot prawn mixture. Serve immediately, with lemon wedges to squeeze over if liked.

nutritional information calories 334 • fat 9 g • saturated fat 1.9 g • added sugar none • fibre 6 g • protein 27.6 g • salt 2.36 g • carbohydrate 38 g

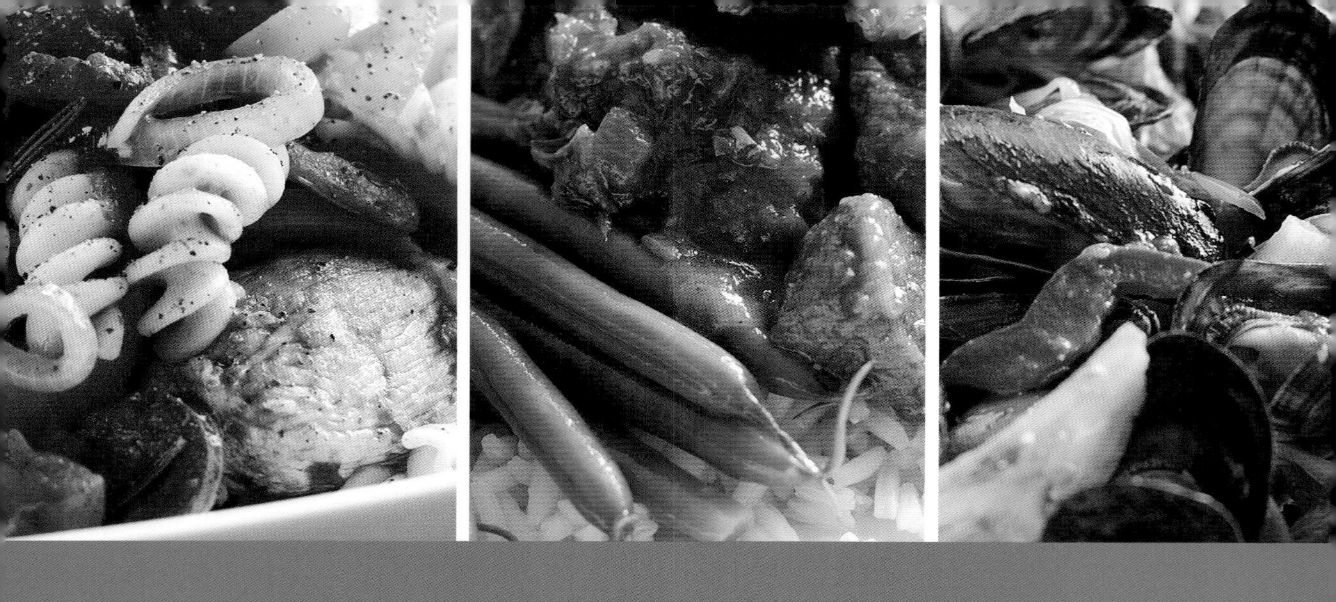

main meals

Whether you're a top-class athlete or a busy office worker you need to eat a rich variety of foods to ensure a balanced diet. However tempting it may be after a hard day's work to come home and put a ready-meal in the oven, for just a little more effort you could be eating one of the delicious recipes featured in this chapter. From fresh fish dishes to spicy suppers and tasty salads, all of these recipes are quick to cook and will help keep you in peak condition.

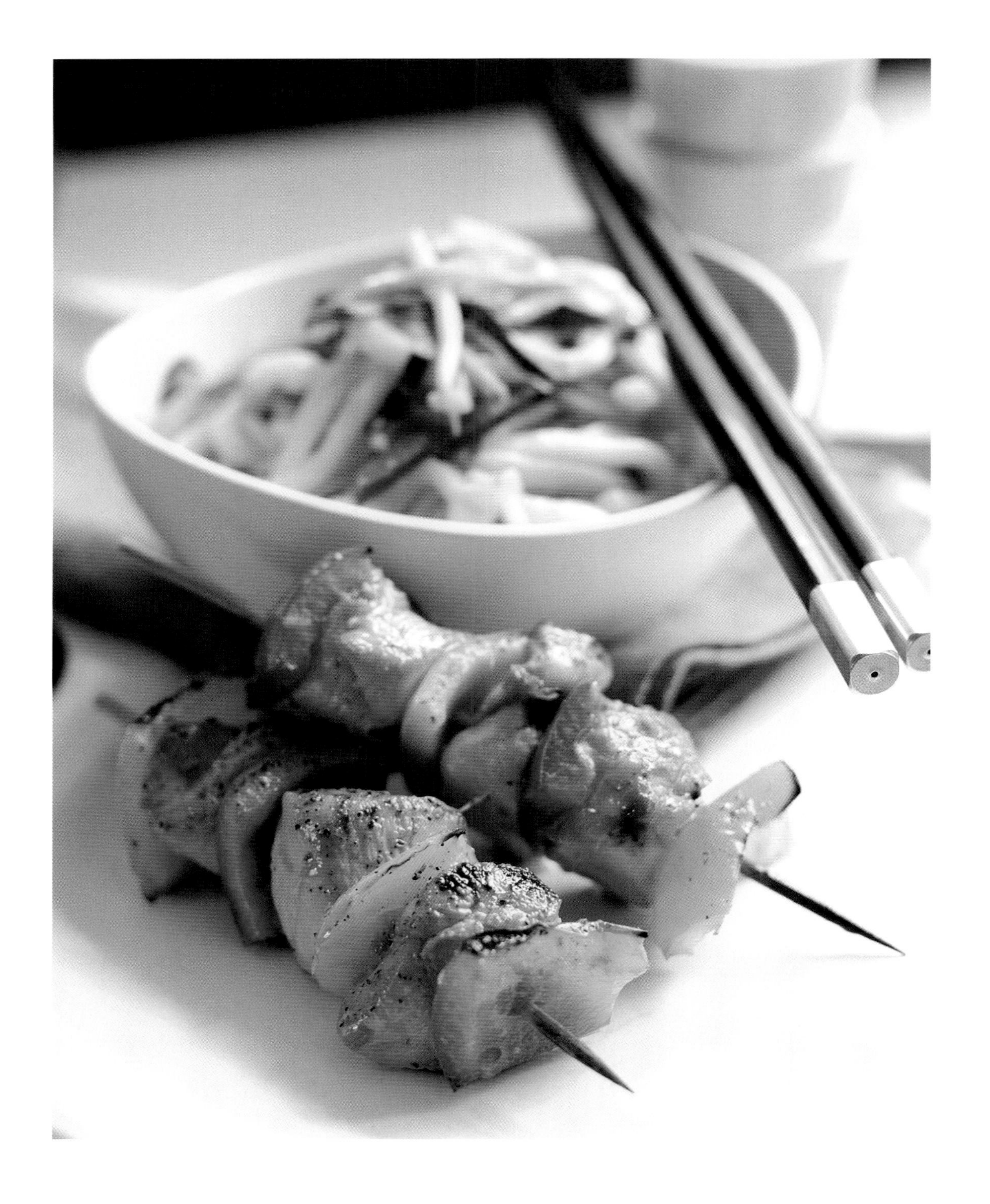

yakitori chicken with udon vegetable noodles

A substantial supper dish, these tasty chicken skewers are good eaten hot or cold. Udon noodles are thick rice noodles – you can get them in the supermarket or a chinese deli. If you can't get hold of them, use flat rice noodles.

4 skinless, boneless chicken breasts
6 tablespoons dark soy sauce
4 tablespoons runny honey
2 tablespoons dry sherry
2 tablespoons minced ginger
1 large green pepper, seeded and cut into chunks
1 large yellow pepper, seeded and cut into chunks
1 tablespoon cornflour
250 g (9 oz) udon noodles
1 tablespoon sesame oil
350 g bag of vegetable stir-fry mix (beansprouts, carrots, cabbage, etc.)

Preparation: 25 minutes plus marinating
Cooking time: 15–20 minutes
Serves 4

- Cut the chicken into the same size chunks as the peppers and toss in a bowl with the soy sauce, honey, sherry and ginger. Cover and leave to stand for 1 hour.

- Meanwhile, soak 8 medium-length wooden kebab sticks in cold water for at least 20 minutes. Preheat the grill to hot.

- Drain the kebab sticks and thread the chicken and peppers alternately on to them. Arrange the chicken skewers on a foil-lined grill pan and grill them for 6 minutes on each side or until the juices run clear.

- Mix the cornflour with the leftover marinade.

- Plunge the udon noodles into a bowl of boiling water. Drain well.

- Heat the sesame oil in a large frying pan or wok and stir-fry the vegetables for 3 minutes. Add the udon noodles and stir-fry for a further 1 minute. Pour over the reserved marinade and stir-fry until hot, thickened and coating the noodles and vegetables. Spoon into serving dishes, top with the yakitori chicken skewers and serve at once.

nutritional information calories 507 • fat 5.1 g • saturated fat 1 g • added sugar 12.1 g • fibre 3 g • protein 40.5 g • salt 4.35 g • carbohydrate 77 g

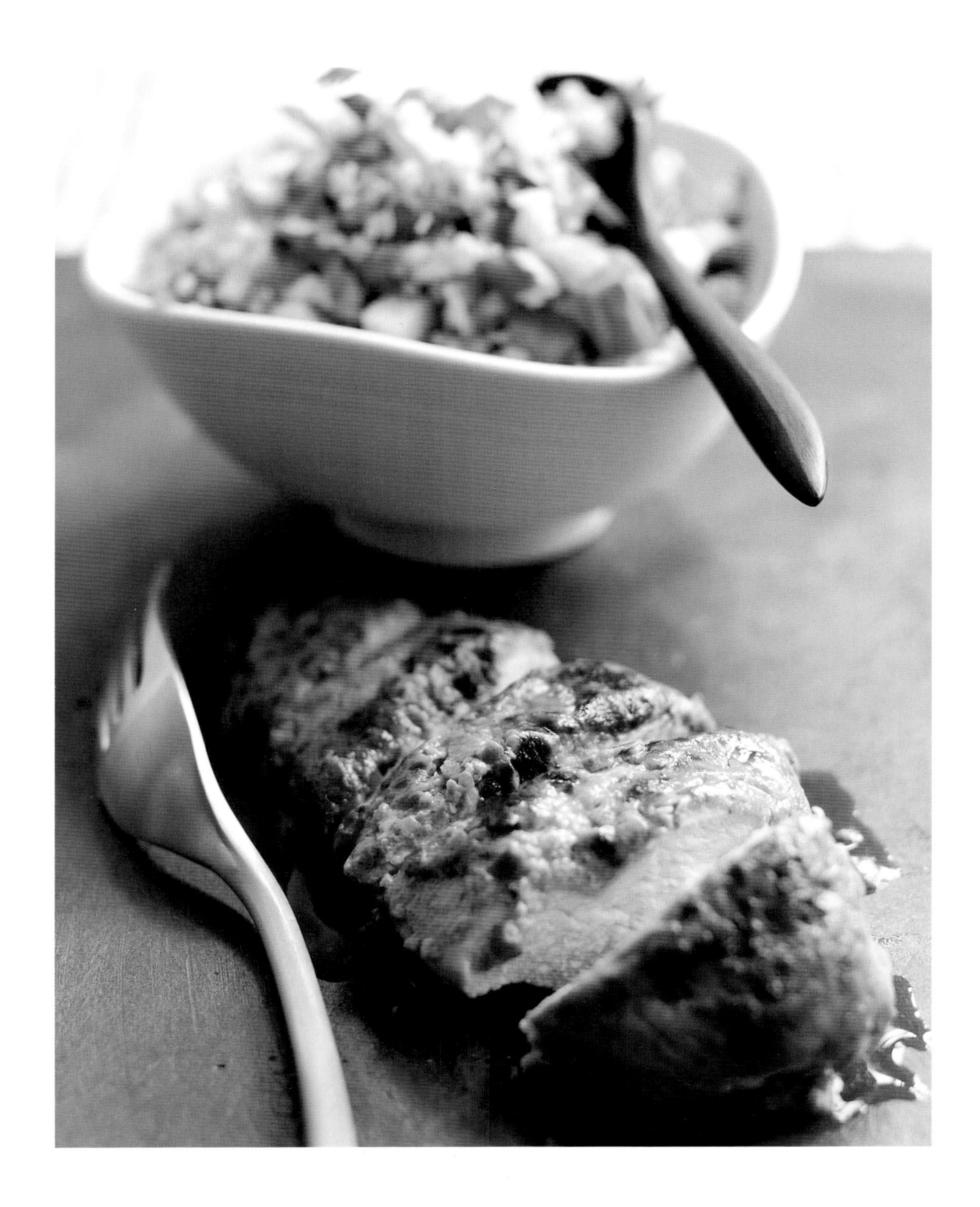

spiced chicken with raita couscous

Hot and spicy and cool and refreshing all in one dish, this is a good after-work recipe for those of you short on time. I always have couscous in my storecupboard – it cooks in minutes: try stirring in some chick-peas for extra texture, protein and carbohydrate.

4 skinless, boneless chicken breasts
200 g tub of 0%-fat Greek-style yoghurt
1 tablespoon curry paste (such as tikka masala, tandoori or madras)
2 teaspoons minced ginger
2 teaspoons minced garlic
juice and finely grated zest of 1 large lemon
175 g (6 oz) couscous
4 vine tomatoes, seeded and diced
4 spring onions, chopped
½ cucumber, seeded and chopped
small handful each of chopped parsley and coriander leaves
salt and freshly ground black pepper

Preparation: 15 minutes plus marinating and soaking
Cooking time: 15 minutes
Serves 4

> Slash the chicken breasts three or four times with a sharp knife. In a shallow bowl, mix together the yoghurt, curry paste, ginger, garlic and half the lemon juice and season with salt and pepper. Add the chicken and turn in the yoghurt to coat. Cover and leave for 30 minutes or overnight.

> Meanwhile, place the couscous in a bowl and pour over enough boiling water to cover. Cover with cling film and leave to soak for 7–8 minutes. Fluff up with a fork and add all the remaining ingredients except the chicken and its marinade. Season well with salt and pepper.

> Preheat the grill to hot. Arrange the chicken breasts on a foil-lined baking sheet and grill for 6 minutes. Turn over, smear with more marinade and cook for a further 8–9 minutes, until beginning to char. Check that the juices run clear and serve with the couscous.

nutritional information calories 313 • fat 3.2 g • saturated fat 0.6 g • added sugar none • fibre 1.6 g • protein 42.8 g • salt 0.73 g • carbohydrate 30 g

chicken, pepper and pasta pot

When in Spain I always eat paella – its rich, spicy flavours are wonderful and I love the tasty pieces of meat and fish that are such a feature of the recipe. This is my version of those robust Spanish tastes. You can make it with rice instead of pasta or serve without either as a casserole and accompany with mashed potatoes.

50 g (2 oz) thin chorizo sausage, thinly sliced
4 small skinless, boneless chicken breasts, each cut into three pieces
1 large onion, sliced
3 garlic cloves, crushed
1 large sweet potato, cut into chunks
leaves from 1 large fresh rosemary sprig
300 ml (½ pint) chicken stock
1 yellow pepper, seeded and thinly sliced
400 g can of chopped tomatoes with chilli
175g (6 oz) fusilli (pasta spirals)

Preparation: 25 minutes
Cooking time: 45 minutes
Serves 4

> Heat a large frying pan, add the chorizo sausage and fry for 1–2 minutes, until the red oil comes out. Add the chicken and cook until browned. Remove the chicken, cover and set aside.

> Add the onion, garlic, sweet potato, rosemary and stock. Bring to the boil and simmer for 5–6 minutes. Return the chicken, add the yellow pepper and pour over the tomatoes. Bring to the boil, lower the heat, cover and simmer for 30 minutes.

> Meanwhile, cook the pasta according to the packet instructions. Drain and stir into the chicken. Serve with crusty bread and a green salad if liked.

nutritional information calories 446 • fat 5.6 g • saturated fat 1.8 g • added sugar none • fibre 5.9 g • protein 41.4 g • salt 0.93 g • carbohydrate 61 g

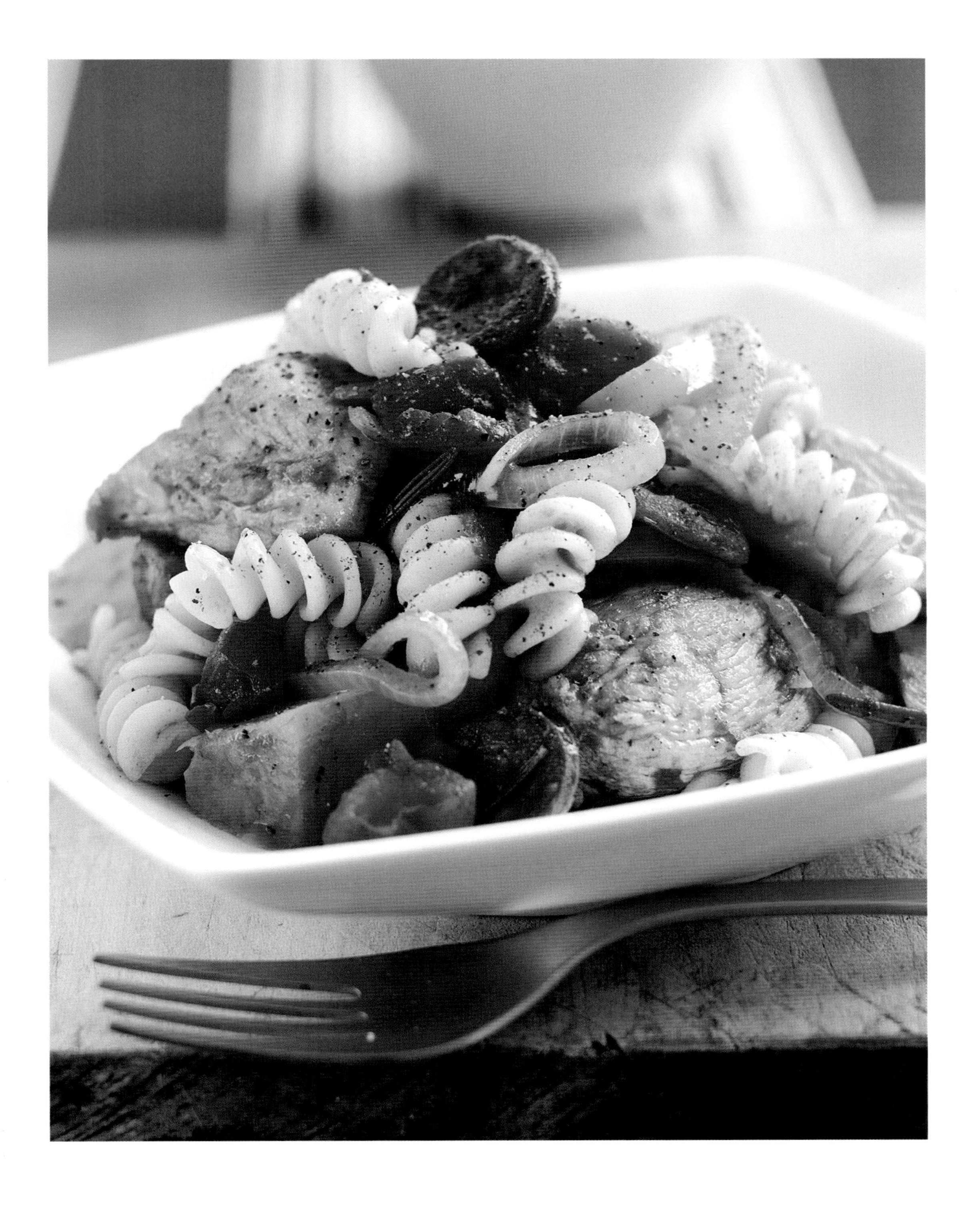

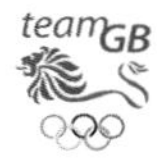

Steve Redgrave's chicken and ham carbonara

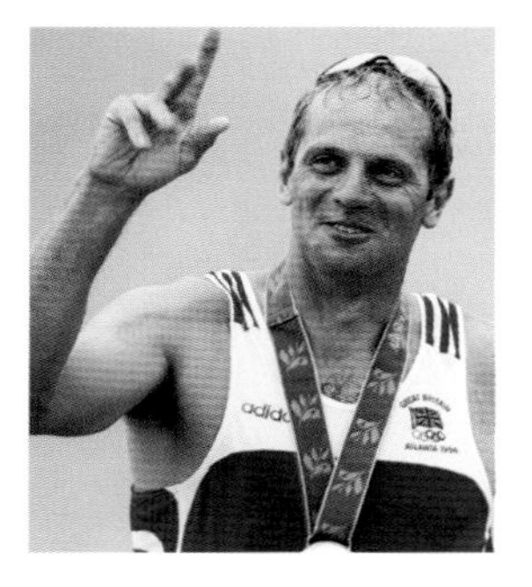

Pasta is one of my favourite foods and contains plenty of carbohydrates, which are so important for any athlete. While I was rowing my calorie intake was around 6,000 a day. Nowadays, however, it is a lot less!

375 g (12 oz) penne (pasta quills)
1 tablespoon olive oil
2 skinless, boneless chicken breasts, cut into small pieces
50 g (2 oz) mangetout, cut into 1 cm (½ in) pieces
4 slices of Parma ham, cut into small pieces
200 ml tub of half-fat crème fraîche
1 teaspoon Dijon mustard
75 g (3 oz) Lancashire cheese, crumbled
handful of flat-leaf parsley
salt and freshly ground black pepper

Preparation: 15 minutes
Cooking time: 12 minutes
Serves 4

> Cook the pasta in plenty of lightly salted, boiling water according to the packet instructions.

> Meanwhile, heat the oil in a large frying pan and fry the chicken over a high heat for 4–5 minutes, until browned. Remove from the pan with a slotted spoon and keep warm.

> Add the mangetout and Parma ham to the pan and fry for 1 minute.

> Return the chicken to the pan, stir in the crème fraîche and mustard and season to taste with salt and pepper. Simmer gently for 5 minutes.

> Drain the pasta and toss with the chicken mixture and Lancashire cheese. Sprinkle over the parsley and serve with warm crusty bread.

nutritional information calories 616 • fat 20.4 g • saturated fat 10 g • added sugar none • fibre 3.2 g • protein 38.6 g • salt 1.6 g • carbohydrate 74 g

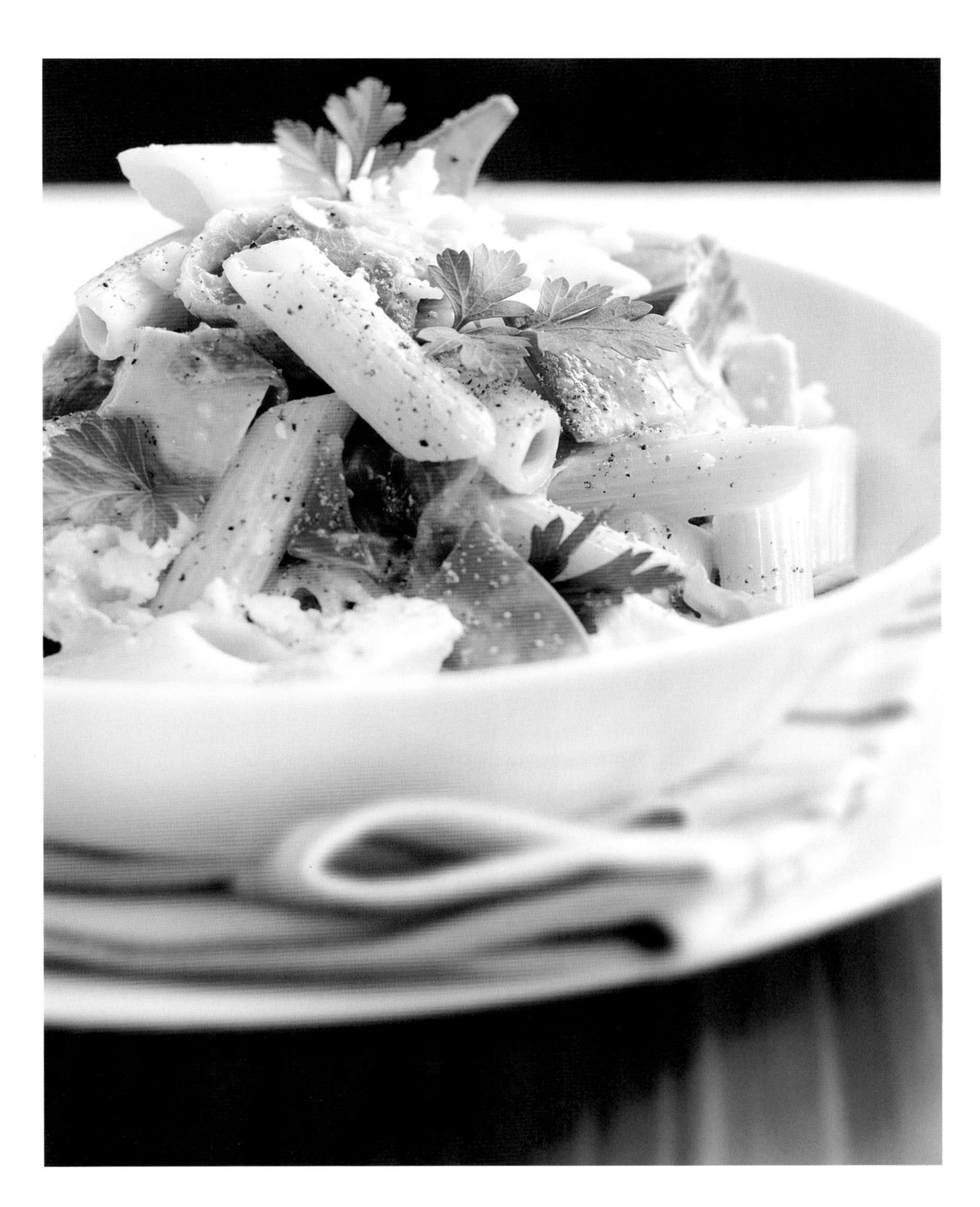

Linford Christie's

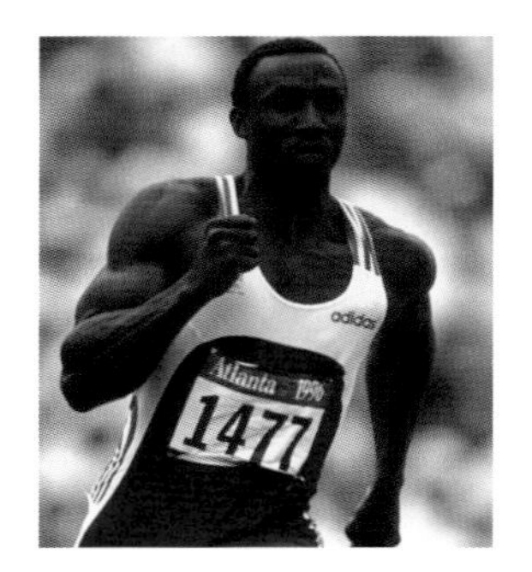

chicken with rice and peas

This is a traditional Caribbean/Jamaican dish that I love. It would usually be made using dried beans but here's the cheat's version – it saves you an hour's cooking time and makes less washing-up! This is the kind of dish that keeps you going all day.

4 chicken thighs, skinned
4 chicken drumsticks, skinned
2 teaspoons chicken seasoning
2 tablespoons Jamaican or medium curry powder
½ teaspoon garlic powder (optional)
1 tablespoon groundnut oil
200 ml (7 fl oz) reduced-fat coconut milk
400 g can of red kidney beans, drained and rinsed
225 g (8 oz) long-grain rice
1 thyme sprig
2 tablespoons cornflour
salt and freshly ground black pepper

Preparation: 40 minutes plus marinating
Cooking time: 1 hour
Serves 4

> Wash the chicken well and then pat dry with kitchen paper. Make a couple of deep slashes through the flesh on each piece. Mix together the chicken seasoning, curry powder, garlic powder (if using) and salt. Toss with the chicken to coat and then set aside – overnight if you have time or for at least 1 hour. This helps to bring out all the different flavours.

> Heat the oil in a large, heavy-based flameproof casserole and fry the chicken for 4–5 minutes until well browned on all sides. Pour over 300 ml (½ pint) water. Bring to the boil, cover and simmer for 30–40 minutes until the chicken is tender.

> Meanwhile, pour 300 ml (½ pint) boiling water into a large saucepan, add the coconut milk. Stir in the beans, rice and 1 teaspoon salt and add the thyme sprig. Bring to the boil, cover and cook over the lowest heat possible for 20 minutes.

> Remove the rice from the heat, cover and leave to stand while you finish the chicken.

> Mix the cornflour with 4 tablespoons water to a smooth paste. Stir into the chicken and simmer for a further 10 minutes. Discard the thyme sprig from the rice and serve with the tender chicken pieces and gravy.

nutritional information calories 557 • fat 14 g • saturated fat 6.6 g • added sugar none • fibre 5.7 g • protein 40.6 g • salt 2.72 g • carbohydrate 71 g

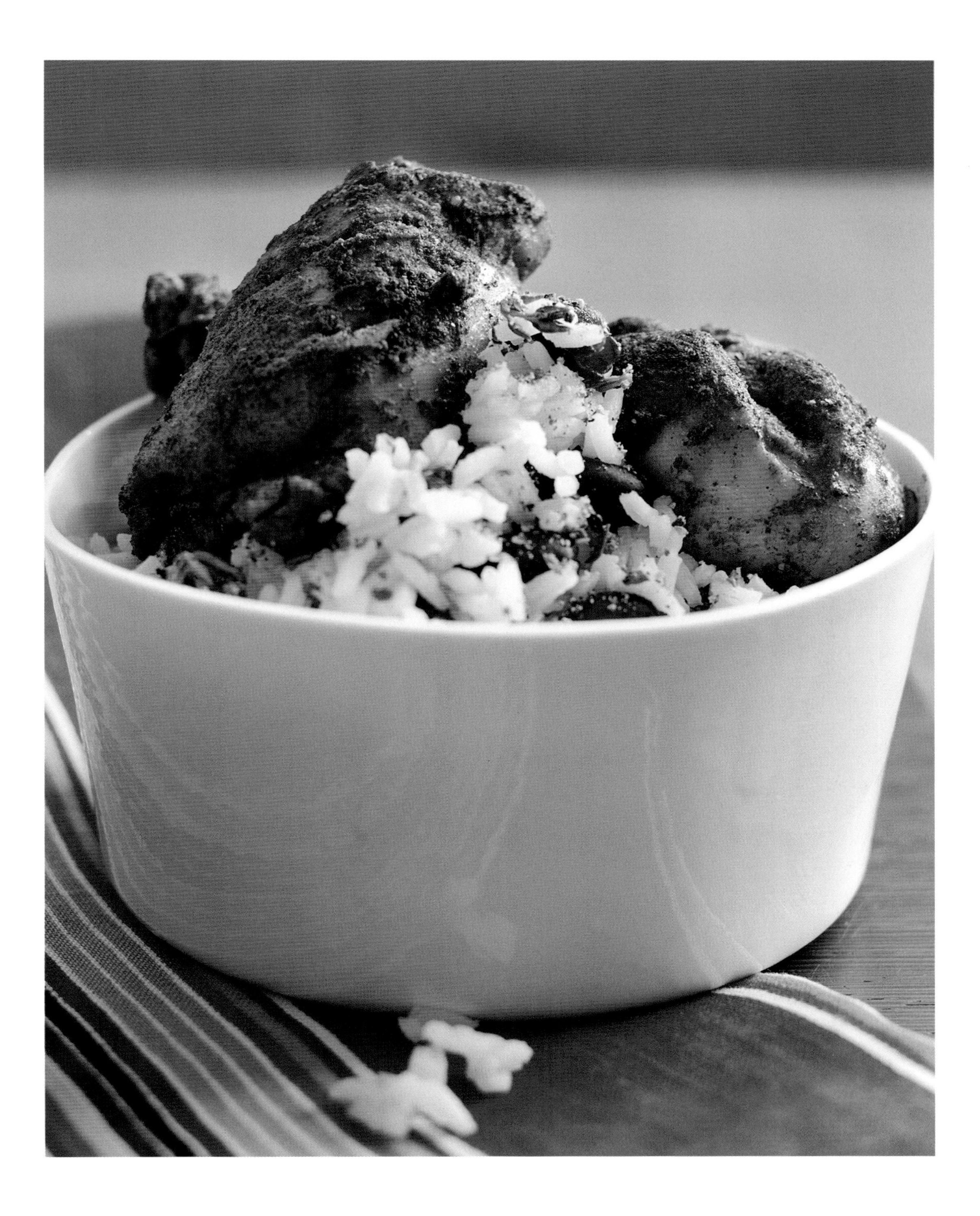

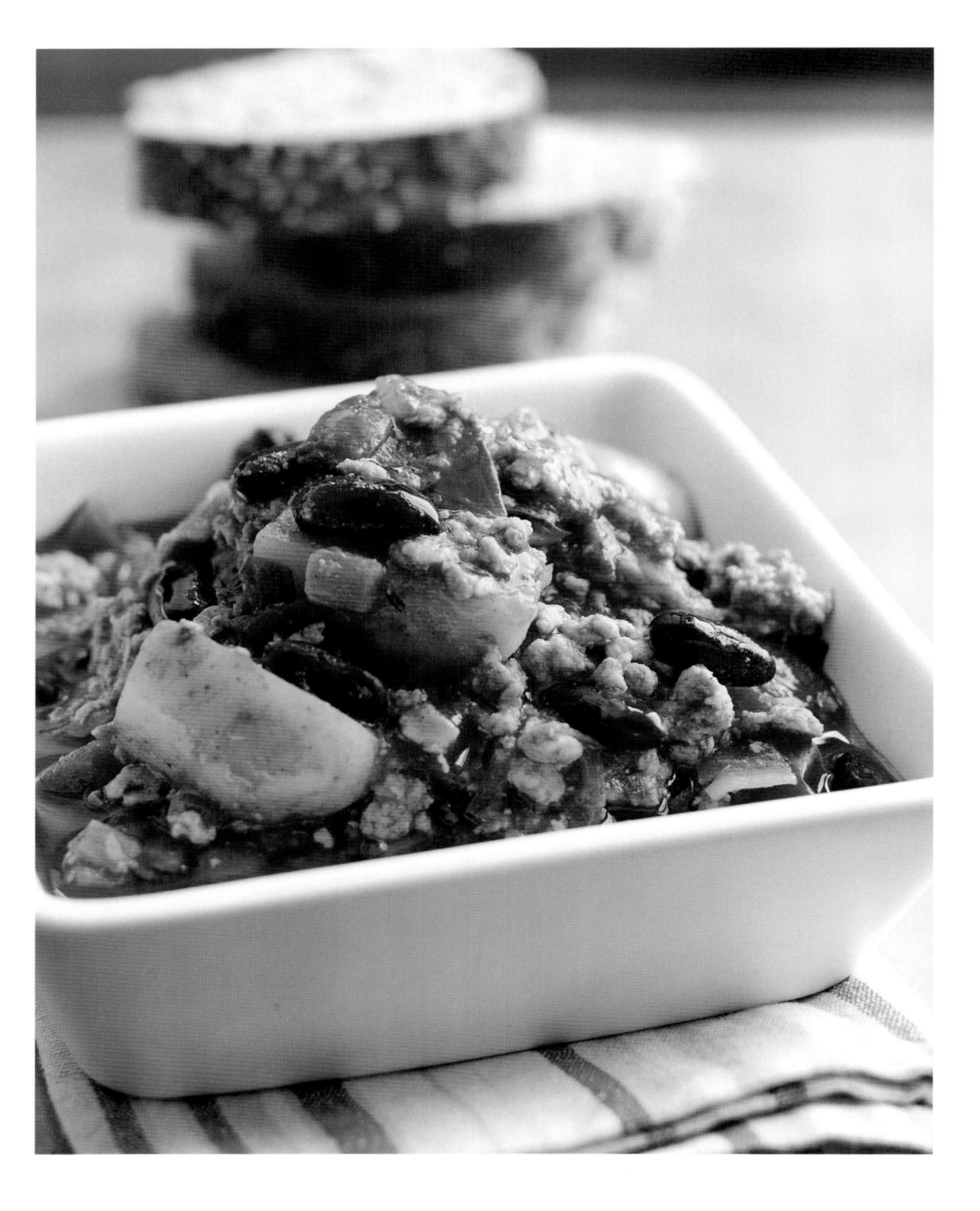

saucy turkey chilli

Turkey is incredibly low in fat and quite inexpensive too. This chilli is a real winter warmer. Omit the chilli and potatoes and you have a superb bolognese mixture – two recipes in one!

1 tablespoon olive oil
1 onion, chopped
500 g (1 lb 2 oz) turkey mince
2 garlic cloves, crushed
2 teaspoons chilli powder
400 g can of chopped tomatoes
2 tablespoons tomato purée
600 ml (1 pint) vegetable stock
1 red pepper, seeded and cut into chunks
450 g (1 lb) new potatoes, cut into chunks
400 g can of red kidney beans, drained and rinsed
150 g (5 oz) baby spinach leaves
salt and freshly ground black pepper

Preparation: 15 minutes
Cooking time: 30 minutes
Serves 4

> Heat the oil in a large saucepan and fry the onion and minced turkey for 4–5 minutes, until the onion is softened.

> Stir in the garlic, chilli powder, tomatoes, tomato purée, stock, red pepper, new potatoes and kidney beans. Bring to the boil, cover and simmer for 20 minutes, until the potatoes are just tender.

> Season to taste and stir in the spinach leaves until just wilted. Serve in bowls, with crackers or warm crusty bread.

nutritional information calories 368 • fat 6.6 g • saturated fat 1.2 g • added sugar none • fibre 8.2 g • protein 39.2 g • salt 2.08 g • carbohydrate 40 g

healthy eating

> Kidney beans and spinach are good sources of iron. Animal protein from the turkey mince in this dish enhances the body's uptake of this essential mineral.

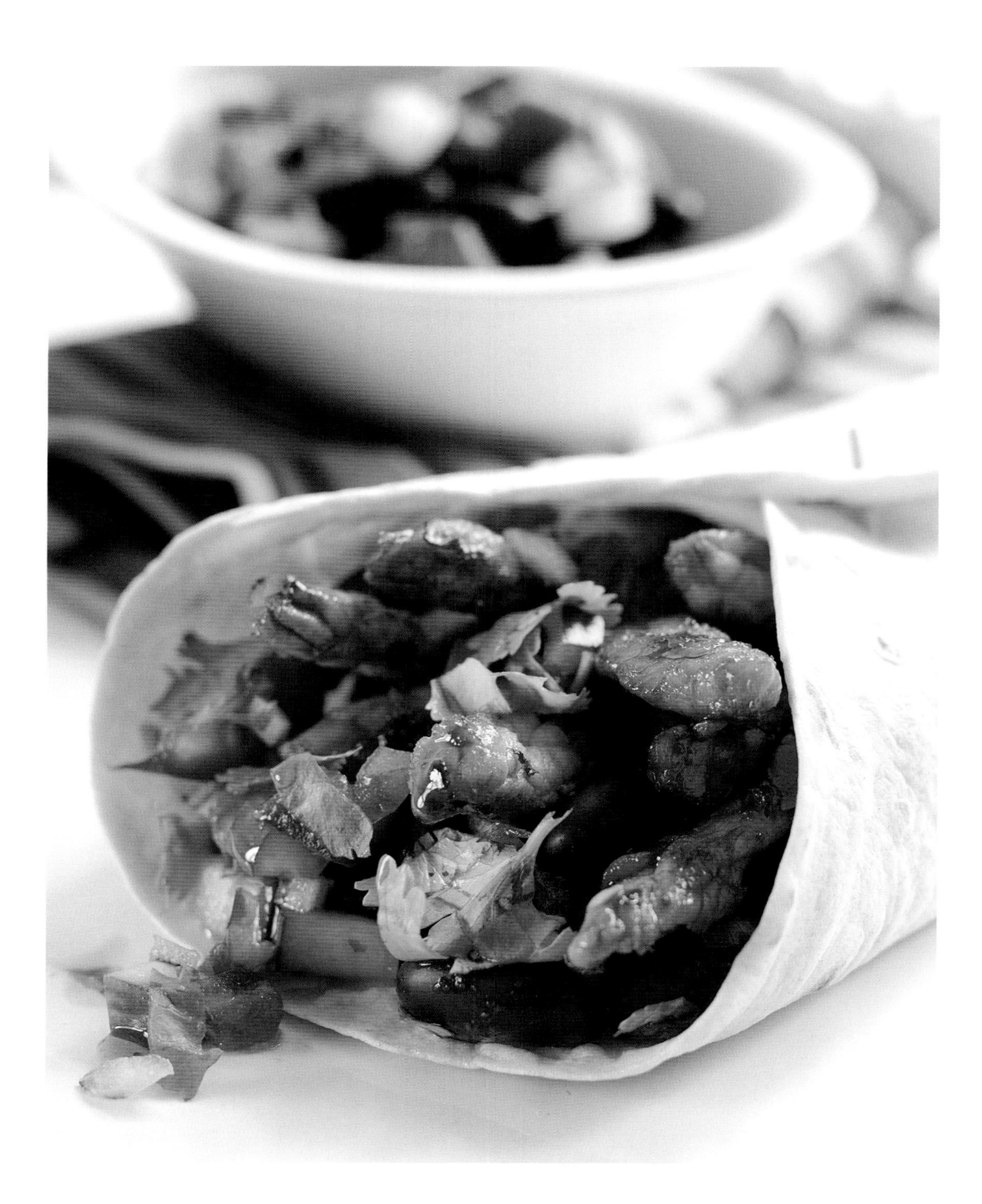

fire 'n' ice tortillas

My kids love this pic 'n' mix or fill-your-own food – it's piled in the centre of the table and we all dive in, which is part of the fun! Use turkey strips instead of pork if you like – these are really low in fat and taste great.

400 g can of kidney beans, drained and rinsed
4 ripe tomatoes, seeded and chopped
1 small red onion, finely chopped
½ cucumber, seeded and finely diced
large handful of chopped coriander leaves
juice of 1 lime
1 tablespoon olive oil
500 g (1 lb 2 oz) pork stir-fry strips
2 teaspoons minced garlic
2 teaspoons minced chillies
2 tablespoons runny honey
8 soft flour tortillas
142 ml tub of low-fat yoghurt
salt and freshly ground black pepper

Preparation: 15 minutes
Cooking time: 10 minutes
Serves 4

> Place the kidney beans in a bowl and break up with a fork or a potato masher. Then stir in the tomatoes, red onion, cucumber, coriander, lime juice and plenty of seasoning to taste.

> Heat the oil in a wok or frying pan and fry the pork over a high heat for 3–4 minutes. Add the garlic, chillies and runny honey and stir-fry for a further 2 minutes, until piping hot.

> Warm the tortillas in a microwave or frying pan and fill with the pork mixture, tomato salsa and a spoonful of yoghurt. Fold over the bottom end of each tortilla (to stop the filling falling out) and roll up.

nutritional information calories 648 • fat 16.7 g • saturated fat 3.3 g • added sugar 8 g • fibre 8.2 g • protein 44.6 g • salt 4.32 g • carbohydrate 85 g

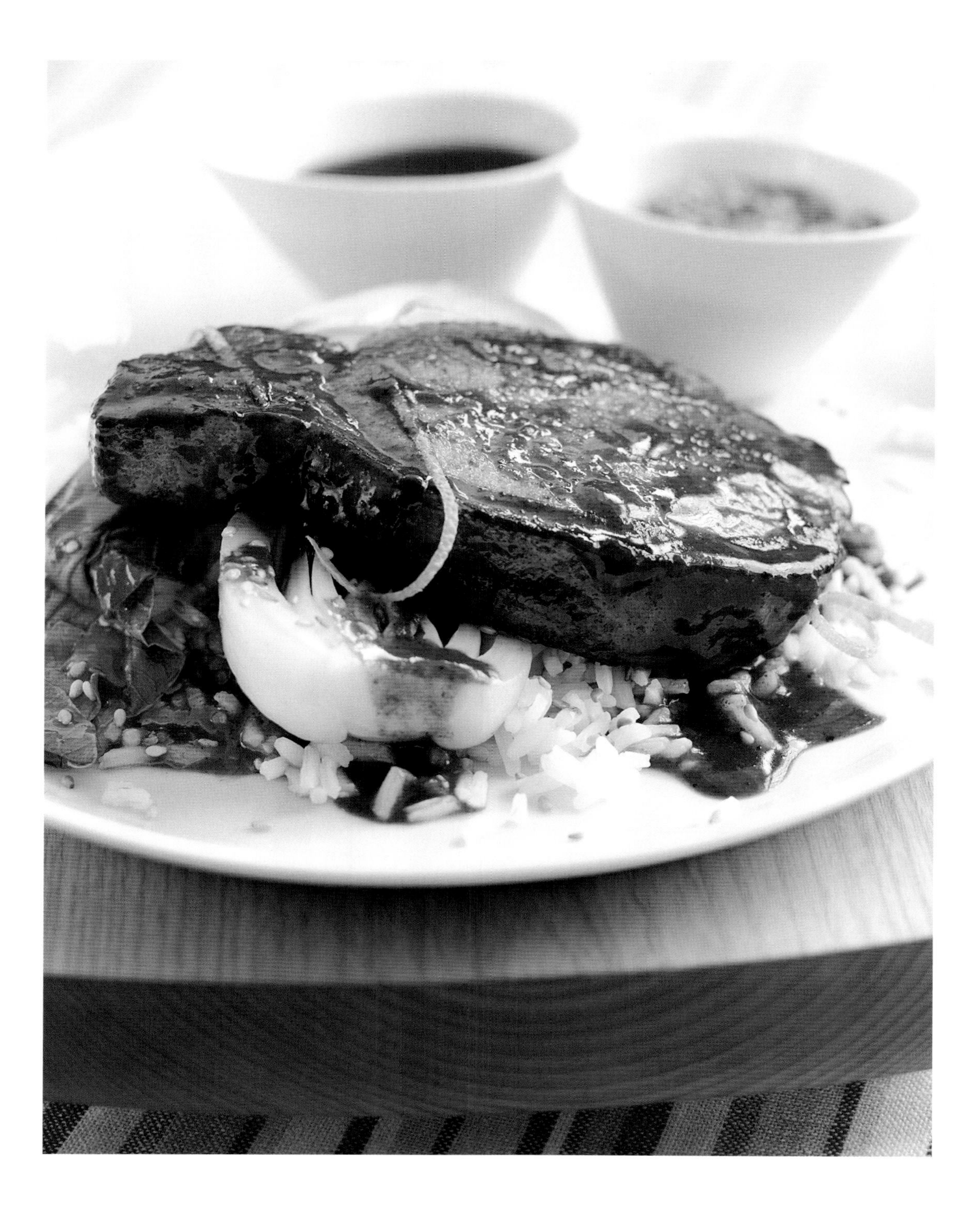

five-spice pork

Simple ingredients create a mouthwatering end result. This citrus marinade works well with pork and any leftover marinade can be warmed through in a pan and drizzled over as a gravy. Loin chops are your best bet for leanness. However, if they do have any fat, just trim it a little.

- 1 tablespoon five-spice powder
- 4 tablespoons hoisin sauce
- 3 tablespoons soft light brown sugar
- 1 tablespoon Worcestershire sauce
- juice and pared zest of 1 orange
- 1 teaspoon minced garlic
- 4 lean loin pork chops, trimmed of all fat
- 225 g (8 oz) long-grain rice
- ½ teaspoon salt
- 4 heads bok choy, halved
- 2 tablespoons sesame seeds, toasted

Preparation: 10 minutes plus marinating
Cooking time: 15 minutes
Serves 4

> In a shallow dish, mix together the five-spice, hoisin sauce, sugar, Worcestershire sauce, orange juice and zest and garlic. Add the pork chops and turn to coat in the marinade. Cover and leave to marinate for 30 minutes.

> Preheat the grill to medium hot. Arrange the chops on a foil-lined baking tray and grill for 15 minutes, turning and basting frequently with the marinade.

> Meanwhile, place the rice, 400 ml (14 fl oz) water and the salt in a large saucepan and bring to the boil. Lay the bok choy over the top, cover and simmer over the lowest heat for 12 minutes, until all the liquid has been absorbed.

> Stir in the sesame seeds and pile on to individual serving plates. Serve with the chops.

nutritional information calories 503 • fat 9.7 g • saturated fat 2 g • added sugar 16.5 g • fibre 0.8 g • protein 38.5 g • salt 1.89 g • carbohydrate 70 g

healthy eating

> Pork is a fabulous source of thiamin, vitamin B1. Thiamin is needed to obtain energy from carboyhdrates, which is vital for exercise.

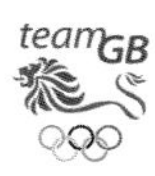

Jonathan Edwards' moroccan lamb

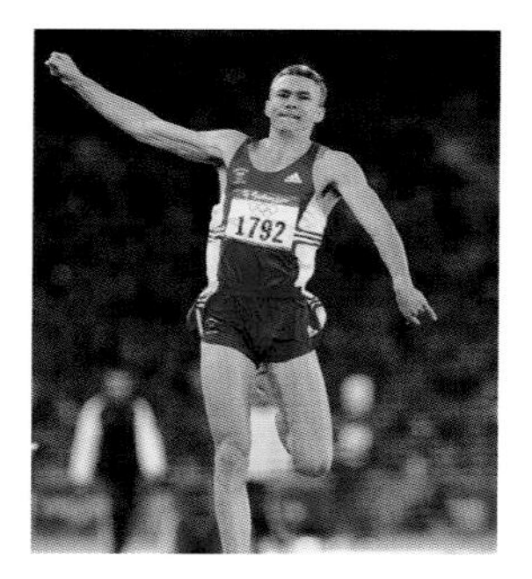

I picked up this recipe on one of my travels around the world to different sports events and have been cooking it ever since. It's not particularly healthy, but, as they say, a little of what you fancy does you good – even if you are an athlete!

½ teaspoon each ground cinnamon, cumin and ginger
750 g (1 lb 10 oz) boneless shoulder of lamb, cut into chunky strips
1 tablespoon olive oil
1 onion, finely chopped
2 garlic cloves, crushed
125 g (4 oz) ready-to-eat dried apricots, quartered
125 g (4 oz) ready-to-eat prunes halved
350 ml (12 fl oz) hot lamb stock
3 ripe tomatoes, roughly chopped
juice and finely grated zest of ½ lemon
small handful of chopped coriander leaves
1 teaspoon harissa paste
salt and freshly ground black pepper

Preparation: 25 minutes
Cooking time: 2 hours
Serves 4

> Preheat the oven to 180°C/350°F/Gas Mark 4. Mix the spices in a large bowl and season with salt and pepper. Toss the lamb pieces to coat them in this spicy mixture.

> Heat the oil in a large flameproof casserole and fry the lamb for 2–3 minutes, until browned.

> Stir in the onion and garlic and cook for 1–2 minutes, stirring well. Add the apricots, prunes, stock and tomatoes and bring to the boil. Cover and transfer to the oven for 1¾ hours or until the meat is tender.

> Remove from the oven and stir in the lemon juice and zest, coriander and harissa. Season to taste and serve with saffron rice and green beans.

nutritional information calories 578 • fat 38.2 g • saturated fat 17.8 g • added sugar none • fibre 4.2 g • protein 36.4 g • salt 0.89 g • carbohydrate 24 g

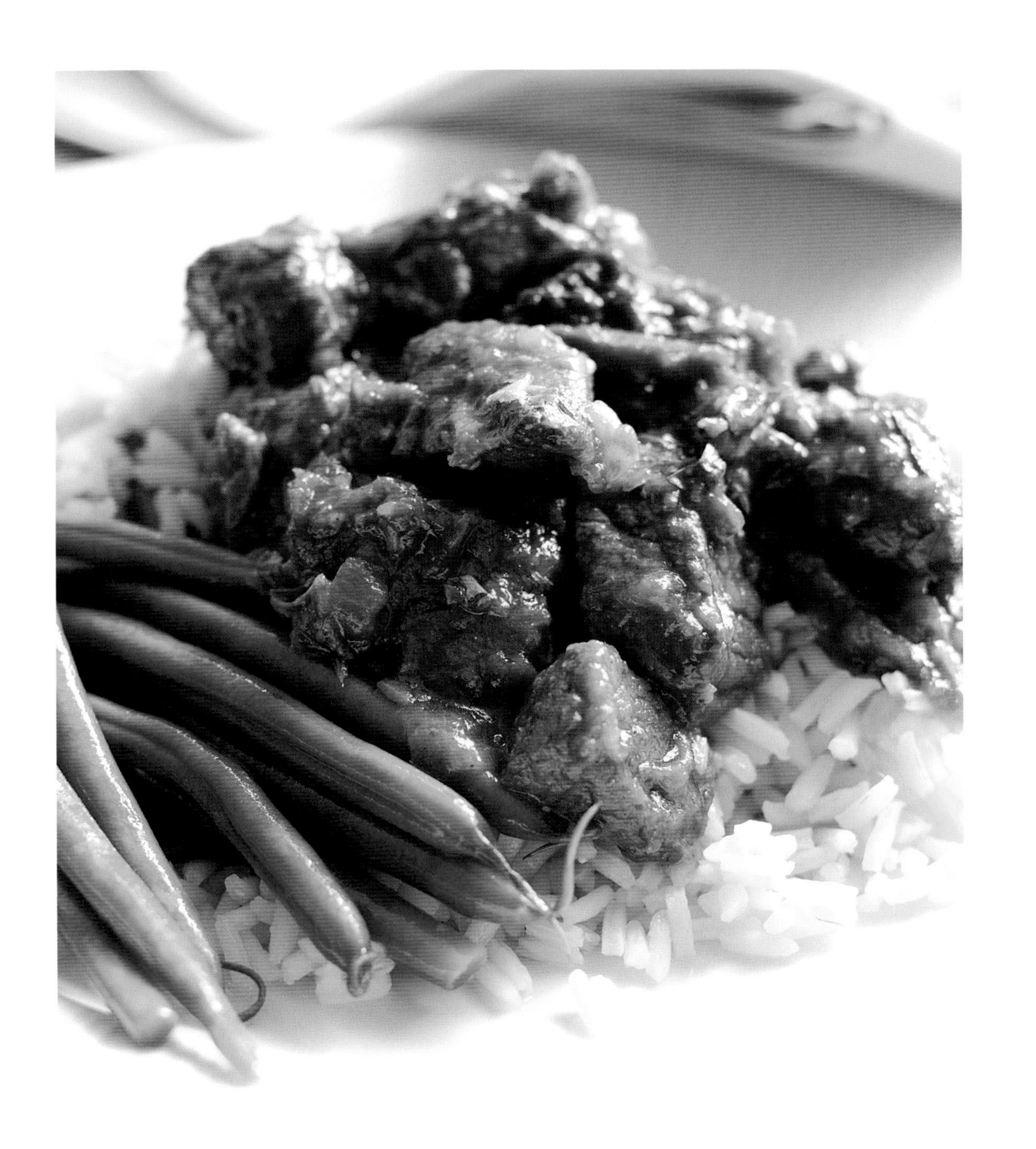

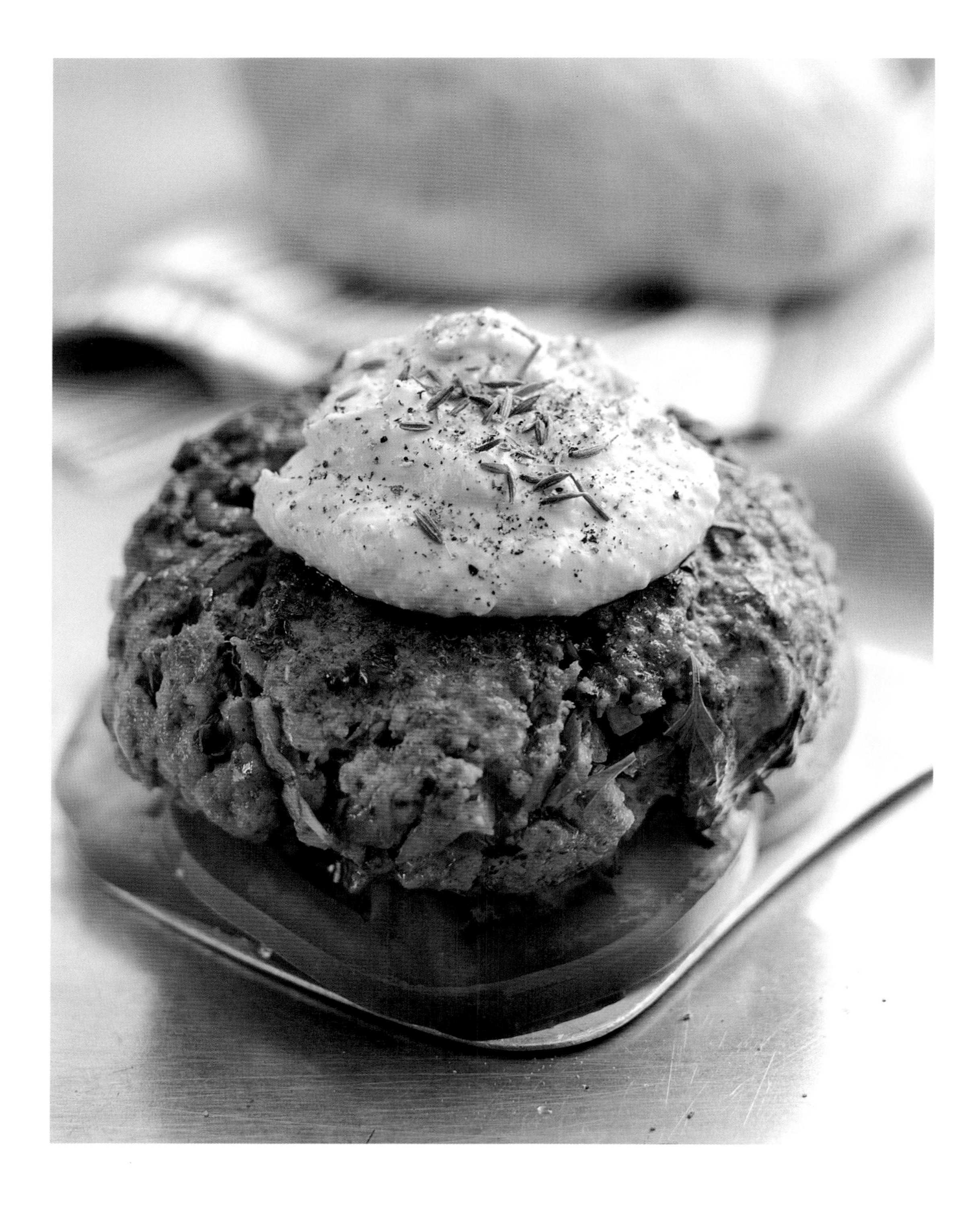

kickin' lamb burgers with houmous

Get your taste buds around this! Juicy burgers that cook just as well outside on the barbie as inside under the grill. Choose your bread – I like to use a tortilla or lavash bread for something a little different, but if you cannot get hold of those, try pitta pockets or crusty ciabatta rolls.

500 g (1 lb 2 oz) lean minced lamb
1 red onion, very finely chopped
1 teaspoon ground cumin
1 teaspoon chilli powder
small handful each of chopped flatleaf parsley and mint
1 tablespoon olive oil
4 tomato tortillas or plain lavash bread
2 large beefsteak tomatoes, sliced
4 tablespoons reduced-fat houmous
½ teaspoon crushed cumin seeds, to serve (optional)

Preparation: 10–15 minutes
Cooking time: 10 minutes
Serves 4

> Mix together the minced lamb, red onion, cumin, chilli, parsley and mint and shape into four burgers.

> Preheat the grill to hot. Brush the burgers with oil and grill for 5 minutes on each side.

> Fold the tortillas or lavash bread into 10 x 25 cm (4 x 10 in) strips. Place some tomato slices in the centre of each tortilla or bread and top with a burger and a spoonful of houmous. Scatter a few of the crushed cumin seeds over the houmous (if using) and serve. Easy!

nutritional information calories 457 • fat 20.4 g • saturated fat 6.3 g • added sugar 1.1 g • fibre 3.1 g • protein 32.5 g • salt 2.07 g • carbohydrate 38 g

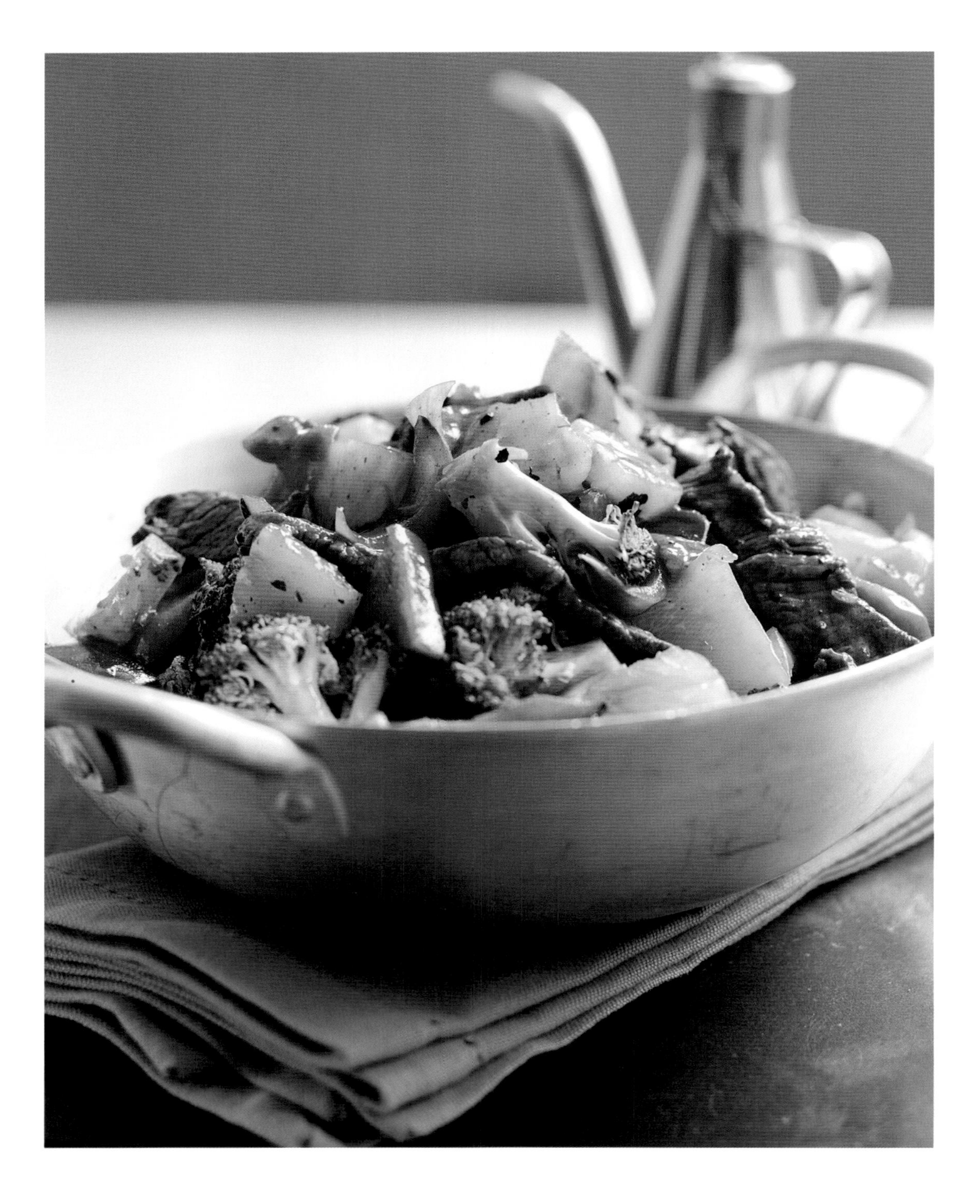

sizzling beef in black bean stir-fry

One of my favourite Chinese dishes that is easy to recreate at home. Choose a lean steak – if necessary, place it between two pieces of plastic film and give it a bash with a rolling pin to flatten it out slightly. I like the fruity addition of the pineapple here, which helps counteract the saltiness of the black bean sauce.

- 300 g can of pineapple slices
- 1 tablespoon vegetable oil
- 350 g (12 oz) lean steak, cut into thin strips
- 2 large red onions, cut into wedges
- 1 large carrot, thinly sliced diagonally
- 350 g (12 oz) small broccoli florets
- 2 teaspoons minced garlic
- 1 red pepper, seeded and cut into chunks
- 1 yellow pepper, seeded and cut into chunks
- 150 ml (¼ pint) black bean sauce

Preparation: 10 minutes
Cooking time: 10 minutes
Serves 4

> Drain the pineapple slices, reserving the juice. Cut the slices into chunks.

> Heat the oil in a wok or large frying pan until hot and smoking, quickly add the beef and stir-fry for 2–3 minutes. Remove with a slotted spoon to a plate, cover and set aside.

> Quickly add the red onions, carrot, broccoli, garlic and pineapple juice to the pan and stir-fry for 3 minutes – the pineapple juice will bubble down to almost nothing. Add the red and yellow peppers and stir-fry for a further 2 minutes.

> Return the beef to the pan, add the pineapple and stir-fry for 1 minute. Pour over the black bean sauce and cook until warmed through. Serve immediately.

nutritional information calories 303 • fat 8.4 g • saturated fat 2 g • added sugar 1.7 g • fibre 6.9 g • protein 28.3 g • salt 2.58 g • carbohydrate 30 g

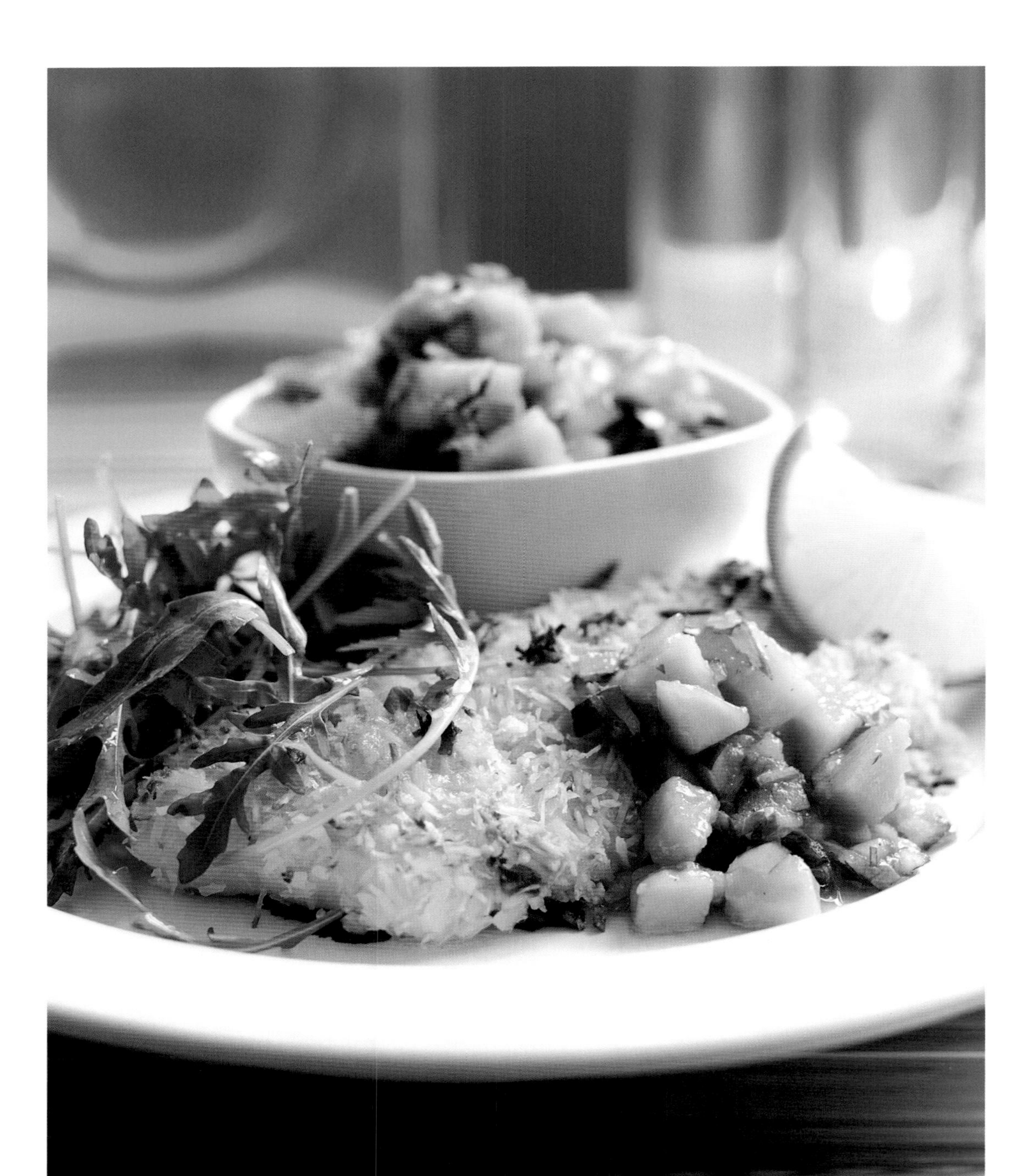

coconut baked fish with papaya and lime salsa

Often the simplest of dishes are the best and this one is no exception – made and on the table in less than 20 minutes. Use your favourite fruits: mangoes, tomatoes or, funnily enough, bananas also work well in this salsa.

- 4 pieces of cod, about 150 g (5 oz) each, skinned
- 4 tablespoons sweet chilli sauce
- 75 g (3 oz) unsweetened desiccated coconut
- 1 papaya, peeled, seeded and cut into chunks
- 1 very small or ½ medium red onion, very finely chopped
- small handful of chopped coriander leaves
- 2 tablespoons lime juice
- 1 tablespoon Thai fish sauce
- 1 teaspoon caster sugar

Preparation: 5 minutes
Cooking time: 12–15 minutes
Serves 4

> Preheat the oven to 200°C/400°F/Gas Mark 6. Dip each piece of fish into 1 tablespoon of chilli sauce to coat, then press into the coconut until evenly covered. Arrange on a baking sheet and bake for 12–15 minutes.

> Meanwhile, combine the remaining ingredients. Mix well and season to taste. Serve with the coconut baked fish and a simple green salad.

nutritional information calories 195 • fat 12.1 g • saturated fat 10 g • added sugar 2.1 g • fibre 4.8 g • protein 8.4 g • salt 1.76 g • carbohydrate 14 g

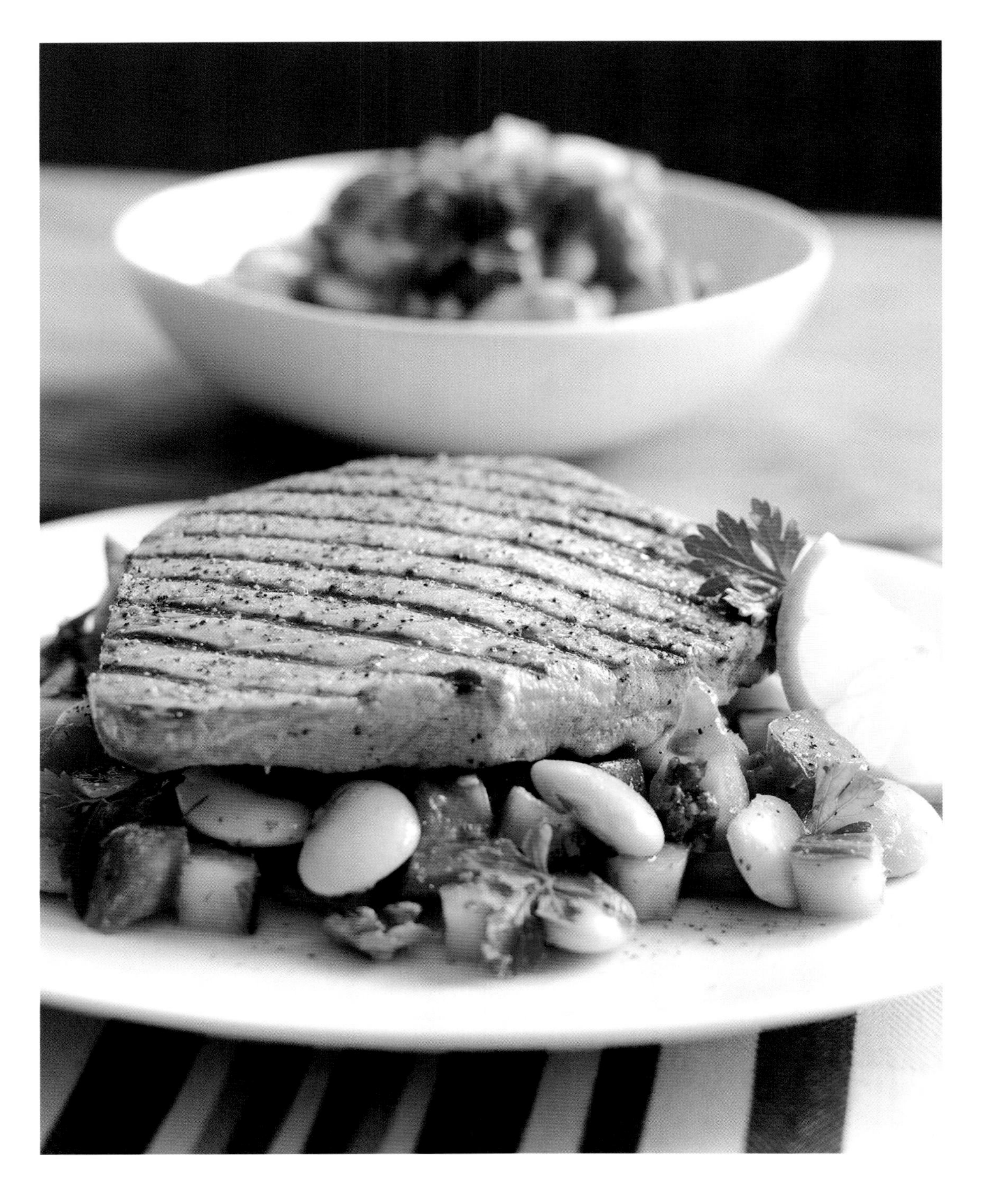

fresh tuna with gremolata butterbean salad

Fresh tuna is beautiful, like a good piece of steak – rich, tender and juicy – and here it is mixed with a flavourful salad. If you closed your eyes you could be on holiday, sitting in a Greek taverna!

2 x 410 g cans of butterbeans, drained and rinsed
3 beefsteak tomatoes, cut into chunks
½ cucumber, trimmed and cut into chunks
1 teaspoon cumin seeds, crushed
1 teaspoon caster sugar
juice and finely grated zest of 1 small lemon
small handful of chopped flatleaf parsley
2 tablespoons olive oil
2 garlic cloves, crushed
4 fresh tuna steaks, about 150 g (5 oz) each
75 g (3 oz) walnut pieces, toasted
salt and freshly ground black pepper
lemon wedges, to serve

Preparation: 10–15 minutes
Cooking time: 5 minutes
Serves 4

> Put the butterbeans in a large bowl with the tomatoes, cucumber, cumin, sugar, lemon zest and half the lemon juice, the parsley and 1 tablespoon of the oil. Toss together and season to taste with salt and pepper.

> Mix together the remaining oil and lemon juice and the garlic and season to taste. Add the tuna steaks and coat well.

> Heat a large griddle pan or non-stick frying pan until hot and smoking. Add the tuna steaks and fry quickly for 2 minutes on each side, until golden.

> Pile the bean salad on to serving plates, scatter over the walnuts and top with the tuna steaks. Serve with the lemon wedges for squeezing over.

nutritional information calories 440 • fat 20.4g • saturated fat 3.5 g • added sugar 1.3 g • fibre 7.2 g • protein 44.2 g • salt 1.69 g • carbohydrate 21 g

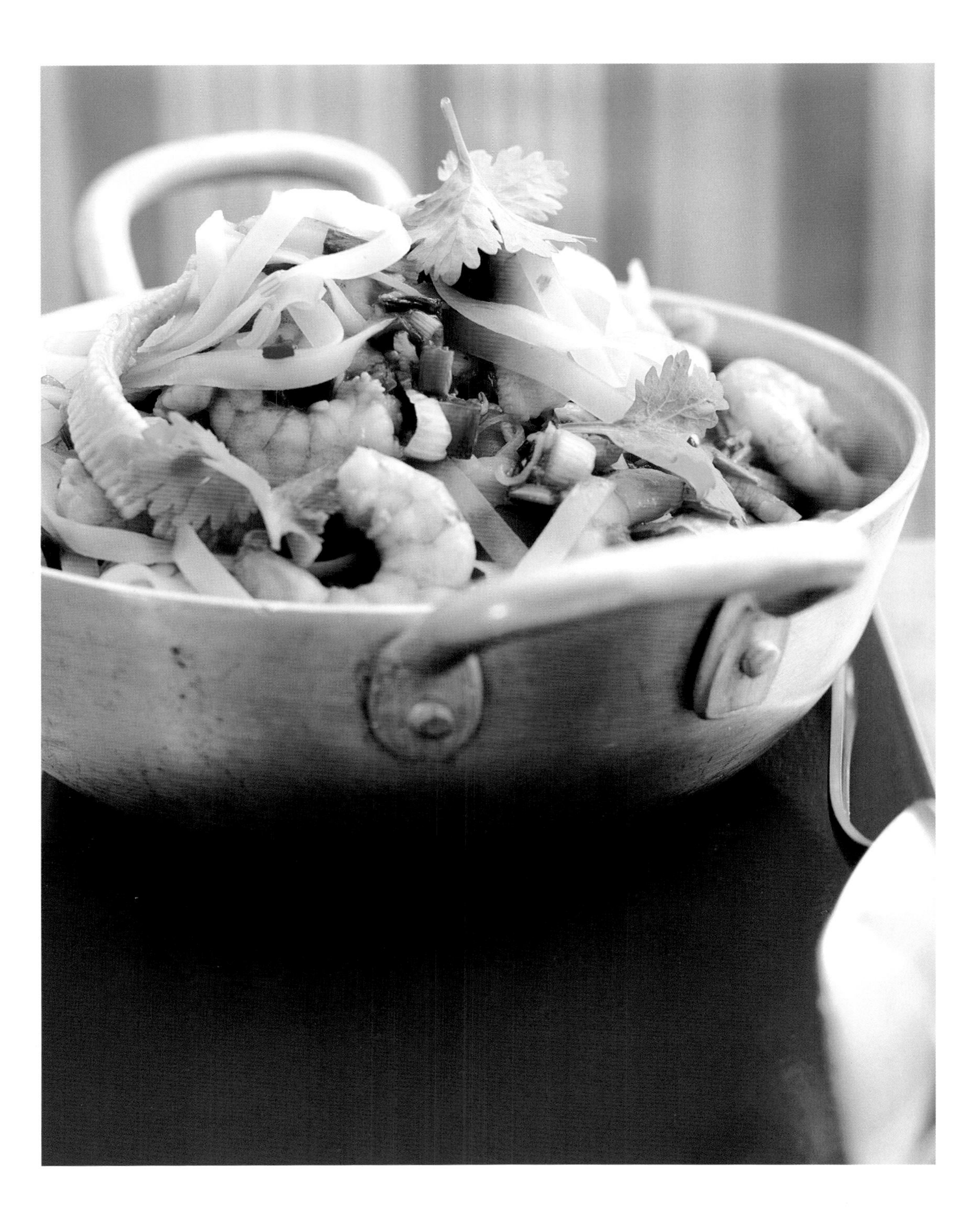

speedy prawn and chilli stir-fry

When you want something quick and tasty a stir-fry always fits the bill and is great for using up all those loose veggies in the fridge. Use chicken instead of prawns if you prefer or, if you are vegetarian, firm tofu.

- 250 g packet of stir-fry vermicelli rice noodles
- 1 tablespoon sunflower oil
- 200 g (7 oz) baby sweetcorn, halved lengthways
- 1 bunch of spring onions, chopped
- 2 teaspoons minced garlic
- 2 teaspoons minced ginger
- 225 g (8 oz) shelled raw prawns
- 2 tablespoons sweet chilli sauce
- 3 tablespoons soy sauce
- juice of 2 limes
- large handful of chopped coriander leaves

Preparation: 5–10 minutes
Cooking time: 10 minutes
Serves 4

> Cook the rice noodles according to the packet instructions.

> Meanwhile, heat the oil in a large wok or frying pan and stir-fry the sweetcorn, spring onions, garlic and ginger for 4–5 minutes until browned.

> Add the prawns, sweet chilli sauce, soy sauce and lime juice and stir-fry until the prawns turn pink and the pan juices have thickened.

> Drain the rice noodles and toss into the prawn mixture, with the coriander. Serve immediately.

nutritional information calories 326 • fat 4.2 g • saturated fat 0.4 g • added sugar 0.6 g • fibre 3.1 g • protein 16.5 g • salt 2.9 g • carbohydrate 59 g

healthy eating

> Stir fries are quick, colourful and a great way to achieve your five-a-day quota of fruit and vegetables, which makes them perfect for athletes.

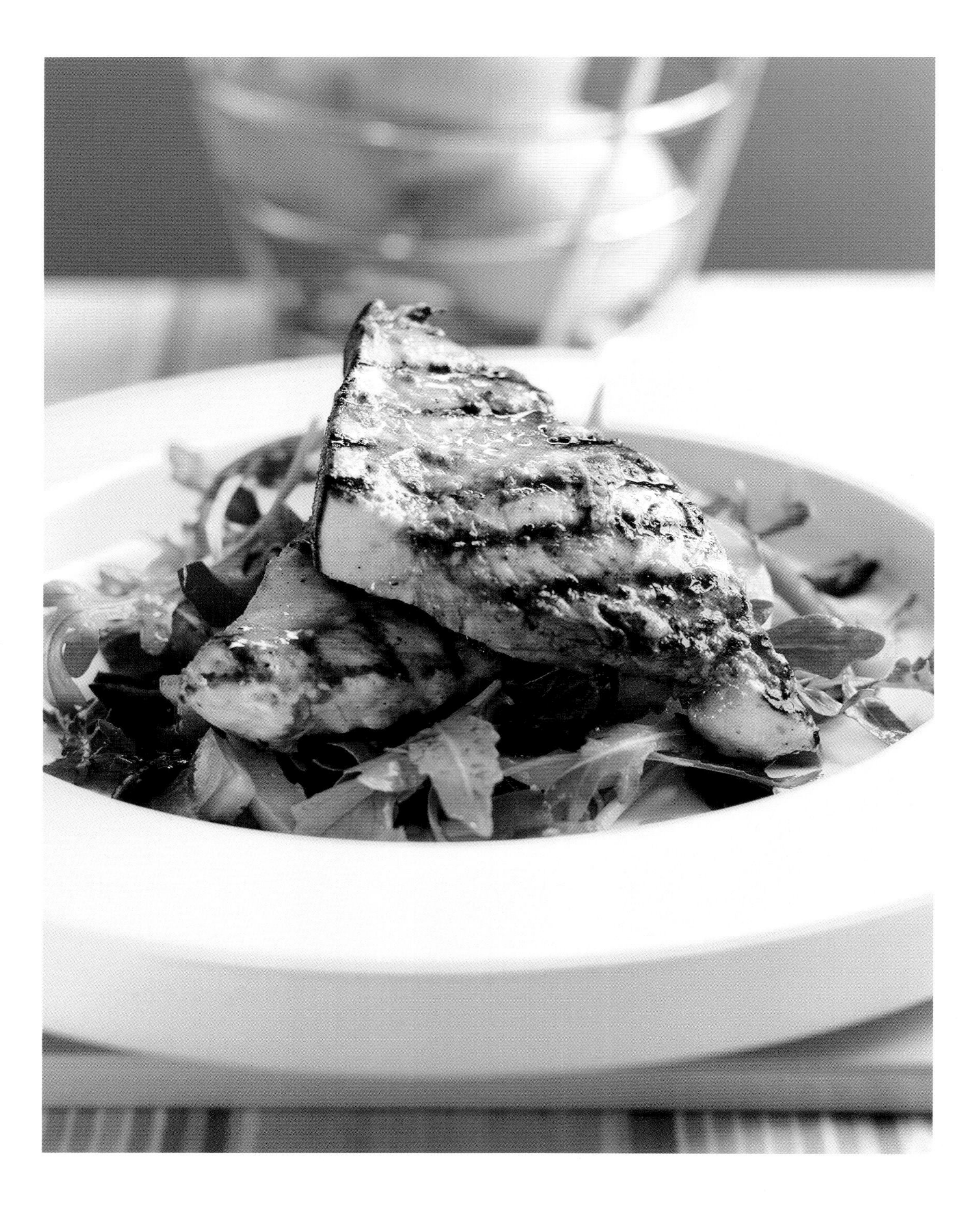

mediterranean swordfish steaks

Swordfish is a little more expensive than cod or haddock – however, for a special occasion it's well worth the extra pennies. If the sun is shining, why not get outside and cook this on the barbecue?

juice and finely grated zest of 1 lemon
juice and finely grated zest of 1 orange
1 tablespoon chopped oregano
4 swordfish steaks, about 175 g (6 oz) each
4 teaspoons olive oil
1 garlic clove, crushed
1 red pepper, seeded and cut into fine strips
1 yellow pepper, seeded and cut into fine strips
2 large ripe tomatoes, peeled, seeded and diced
50 g (2 oz) pitted black olives, quartered
2 oranges, segmented
50 g bag of wild rocket
freshly ground black pepper

Preparation: 10 minutes plus marinating
Cooking time: 8–10 minutes
Serves 4

> Place the lemon and orange zest and juice in a large, shallow dish and stir in the oregano and plenty of black pepper. Cut the swordfish steaks in half diagonally and turn in the marinade to coat. Leave at room temperature for 1 hour to marinate.

> Lift the fish out of the marinade and use 2 teaspoons of the olive oil to brush over both sides of the fish.

> Heat a large griddle pan until smoking and hot and cook the fish for 1 minute, rotate to scorch lines in the opposite direction and cook for a further minute. Turn over and repeat on the other side. Then remove from the heat and leave on the griddle.

> Heat the remaining oil in a large wok or frying pan and fry the garlic and red and yellow peppers for 2 minutes. Pour over any remaining marinade and bubble until hot. Remove from the heat and stir in the tomatoes, olives and oranges. Arrange on four serving plates and scatter over the rocket leaves. Lay two pieces of fish on top of each and serve immediately.

nutritional information calories 304 • fat 12.1 g • saturated fat 2 g • added sugar none • fibre 3.8 g • protein 34.5 g • salt 1.33 g • carbohydrate 15 g

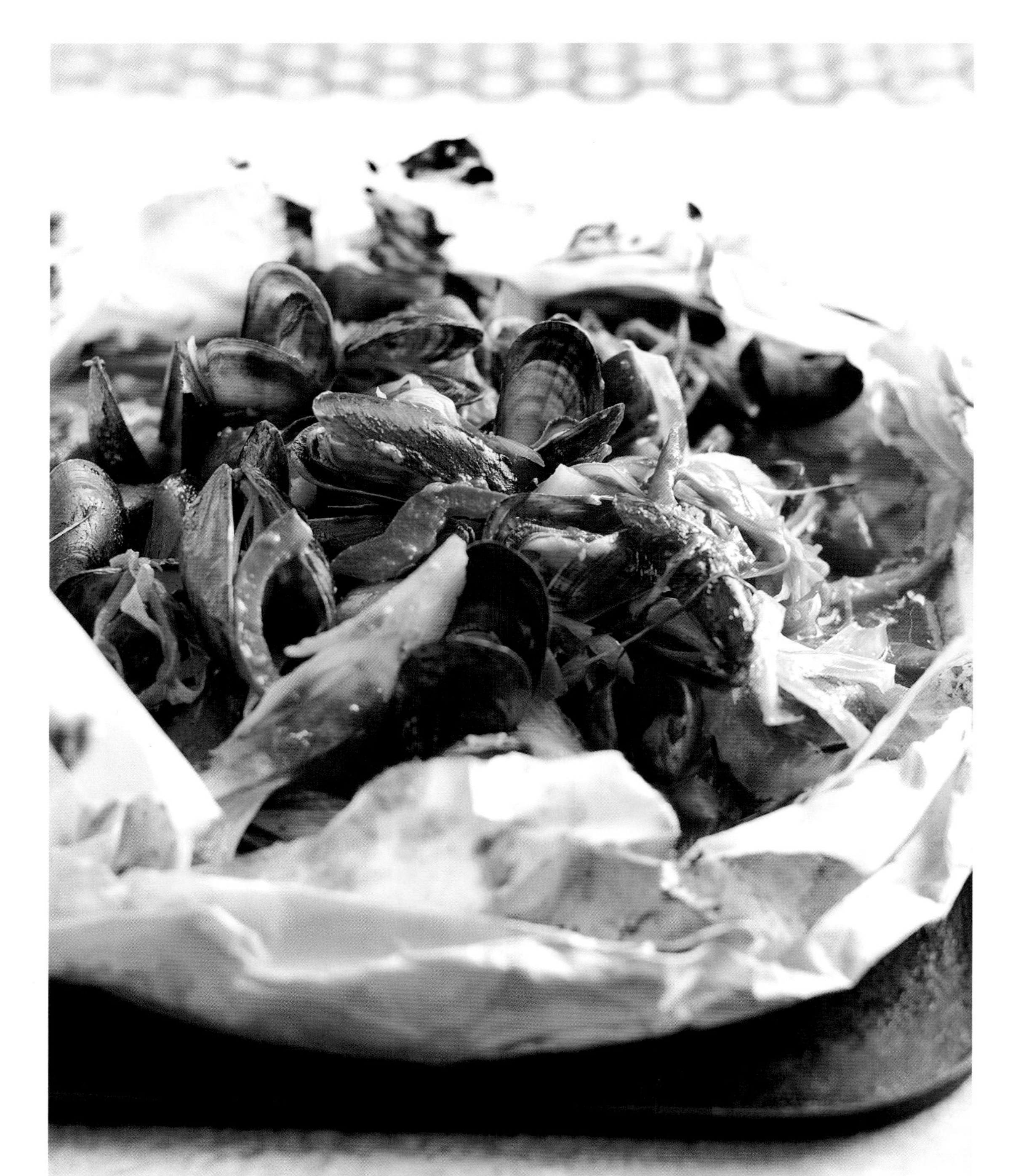

mussels in a bag

Buy ready-cleaned mussels in a net bag – they're plentiful between the months of September and April and they're cheap. Add a few ingredients and – hey presto! – a one-pot meal ready in minutes.

- 1.5 kg (3 lb 5 oz) fresh ready-cleaned black mussels
- 1 tablespoon olive oil
- 2 garlic cloves crushed
- 4 spring onions, shredded
- 1 red pepper, seeded and cut into thin strips
- 1 fennel bulb, trimmed, halved and thinly sliced
- 1 teaspoon minced chillies
- 5 tablespoons Szechuan spicy tomato sauce

Preparation: 15 minutes
Cooking time: 15 minutes
Serves 4

> Preheat the oven to 230°C/450°F/Gas Mark 8. Rinse the mussels in cold water and discard any that are damaged or that are open and do not close when sharply tapped. Pull out any beards and pat the mussels dry with kitchen paper.

> Tear a large piece of greaseproof paper and fold in half to make a square large enough to hold the mussels. Open up the paper and set aside.

> Heat the oil in a large wok and stir-fry the garlic, spring onions, red pepper, fennel and minced chillies for 1–2 minutes, until just beginning to soften. Tip in the mussels and Szechuan sauce and stir. Pile into the centre of one half of the paper. Fold over and pinch the edges together to seal. Place on a baking sheet and bake for 10–12 minutes.

> Tear open the bag and serve immediately, with crusty bread, if liked.

nutritional information calories 139 • fat 5.5 g • saturated fat 0.7 g • added sugar 0.8 g • fibre 1.7 g • protein 14.9 g • salt 0.99 g • carbohydrate 8 g

“ It was vital that I maintained my energy levels for training and racing. ” > **Linford Christie**

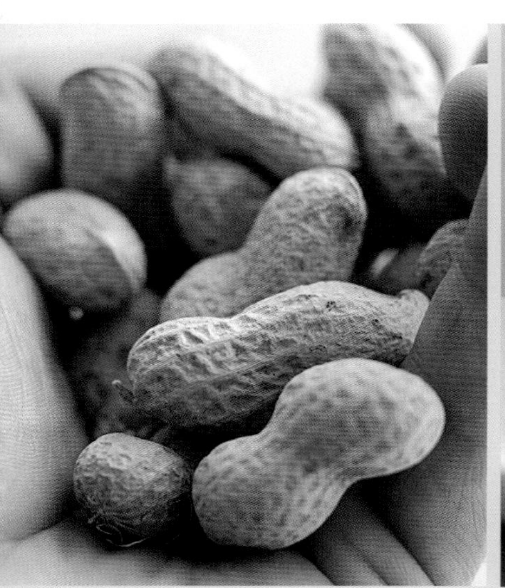

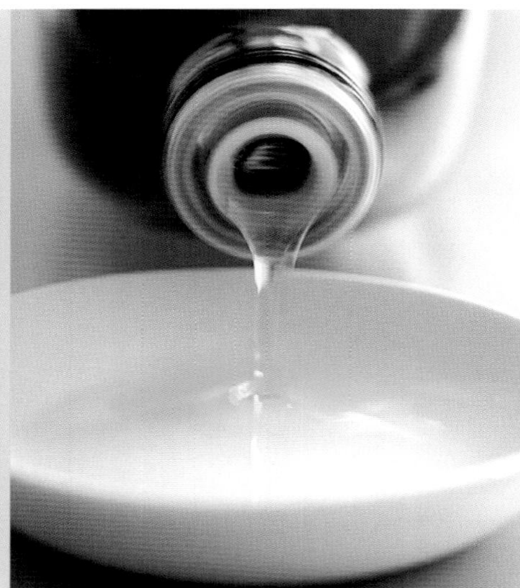

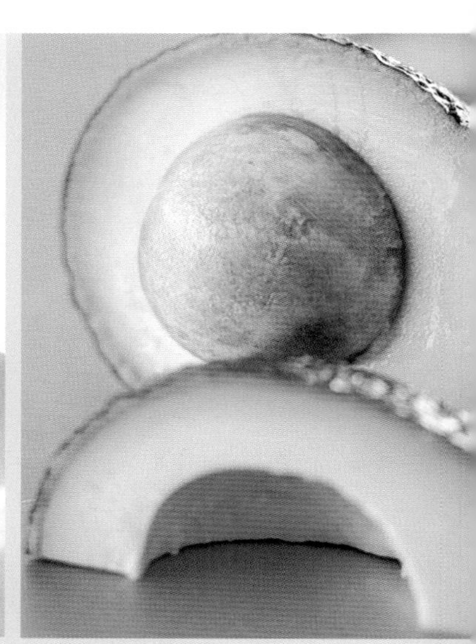

HIGHER FAT CHOICE	LOWER FAT CHOICE
full-fat milk	semi-skimmed and skimmed milk
creamed coconut	lower-fat coconut milk
ice-cream	sorbet
chicken with skin	chicken without skin
streaky bacon	back bacon, trimmed
cheese	reduced-fat cheese
crisps	pretzels
thin-cut chips	thick-cut chips

An Olympic sprinter with 23 major championships to his name, Linford Christie needed a diet to bring his body to peak condition time and time again. Sprinting is about converting pure power into speed and this means having plenty of lean muscle and not carrying too much body fat. Controlling his body weight and body fat was therefore vital to his performance.

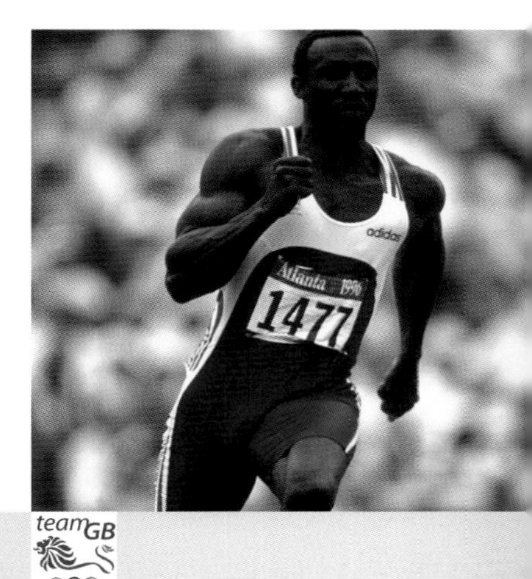

fats and oils

teamGB

Linford needed carefully timed meals and snacks before and after training so that his muscles would have the fuel necessary to repair, grow and respond to the training. Where every meal and snack counted, overeating fried and fatty foods would have resulted in unwanted weight gain and slower times. Every gram of fat provides 9kcal yet carbohydrate and protein provide 4kcal, so by focusing his meals around a balance of carbohydrate and protein-rich foods and by keeping his fat intake low, weight management could be achieved.

His diet was not fat-free, however, and neither should yours be. Some fats are essential to health – for skin, hair and eyes as well as for hormones and the immune system. Good sources of essential fats are found in oily fish such as trout and salmon, in nuts, seeds, avocados and small amounts of vegetable oil.

Looking at his food diary, we can see that Linford used a variety of ways to keep his fat intake, and his weight, in check; some are listed in the table, left. Despite superhuman achievements, even Linford had the occasional high-fat meal or snack – but it is what he ate 90 per cent of the time that made the difference.

Linford's food diary

> **Breakfast**

Porridge made with cornmeal, oats and banana (mother's recipe) and a cup of normal or herbal tea.

> **Lunch**

Preferred to snack on fruit.

> **Main meal**

Big meal of West Indian chicken or fish with rice, broccoli and carrots. Preferred white meat and fish to red meat.

> **In between**

I loved snacking on all types of fruit, such as mangoes, grapes, satsumas, plums, oranges, bananas and all types of berry.

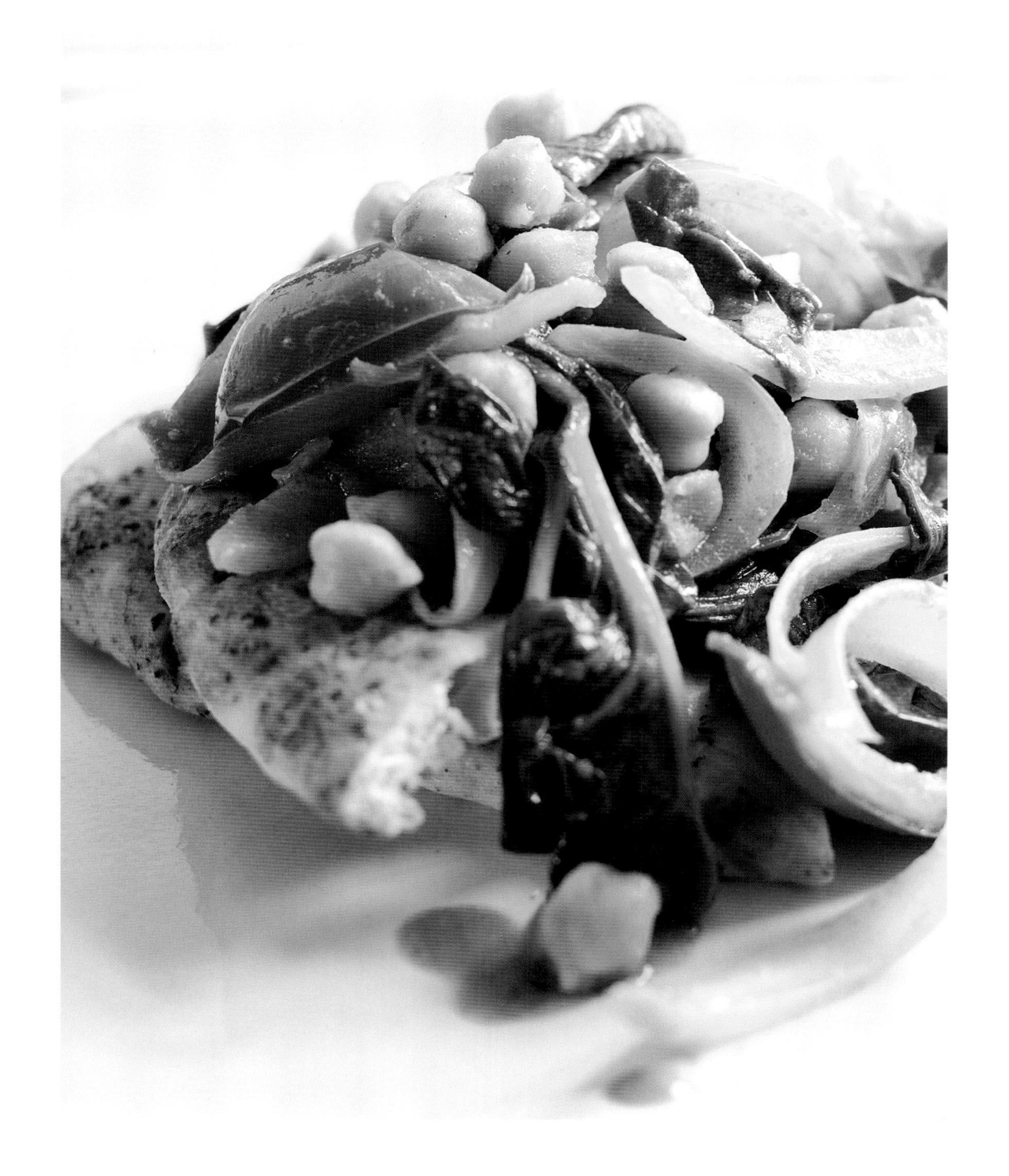

spicy beans on toast

Almost everyone loves beans on toast! They are quick, easy and nutritious. Here is a spicy variation with an Indian feel for those days when you feel like something a bit special – even easier than a takeaway and much more healthy.

- 1 tablespoon vegetable oil
- 1 large onion, cut into thin wedges
- 1 teaspoon ground turmeric
- 1 teaspoon ground cumin
- 3 tomatoes, seeded and cut into wedges
- 400 g can of chick-peas, drained and rinsed
- 4 mini garlic and coriander naan breads
- 125 g (4 oz) baby spinach leaves
- handful of coriander leaves
- chopped coriander, to serve (optional)

Preparation: 5 minutes
Cooking time: 15 minutes
Serves 4

> Heat the oil in a frying pan. Add the onion and fry over a low heat for 5–6 minutes. Add the turmeric and cumin and cook for a further 2–3 minutes, until softened and golden. Add the tomatoes, chick-peas and 4 tablespoons water and heat through for a minute or so.

> Pop the naan bread into a toaster to warm through and then cut in half and arrange two pieces on each plate.

> Stir the spinach into the bean mixture and cook until just wilted. Spoon over the naan bread. Scatter with fresh coriander and serve each portion with a wedge of lemon to squeeze over.

nutritional information calories 275 • fat 7.3 g • saturated fat 1.3 g • added sugar 0.6 g • fibre 5.6 g • protein 10.7 g • salt 1.41 g • carbohydrate 44 g

healthy eating

> Chick-peas are a great source of protein and fibre, plus they are low in fat. Canned chick-peas should be drained and rinsed before use to get rid of any excess salt.

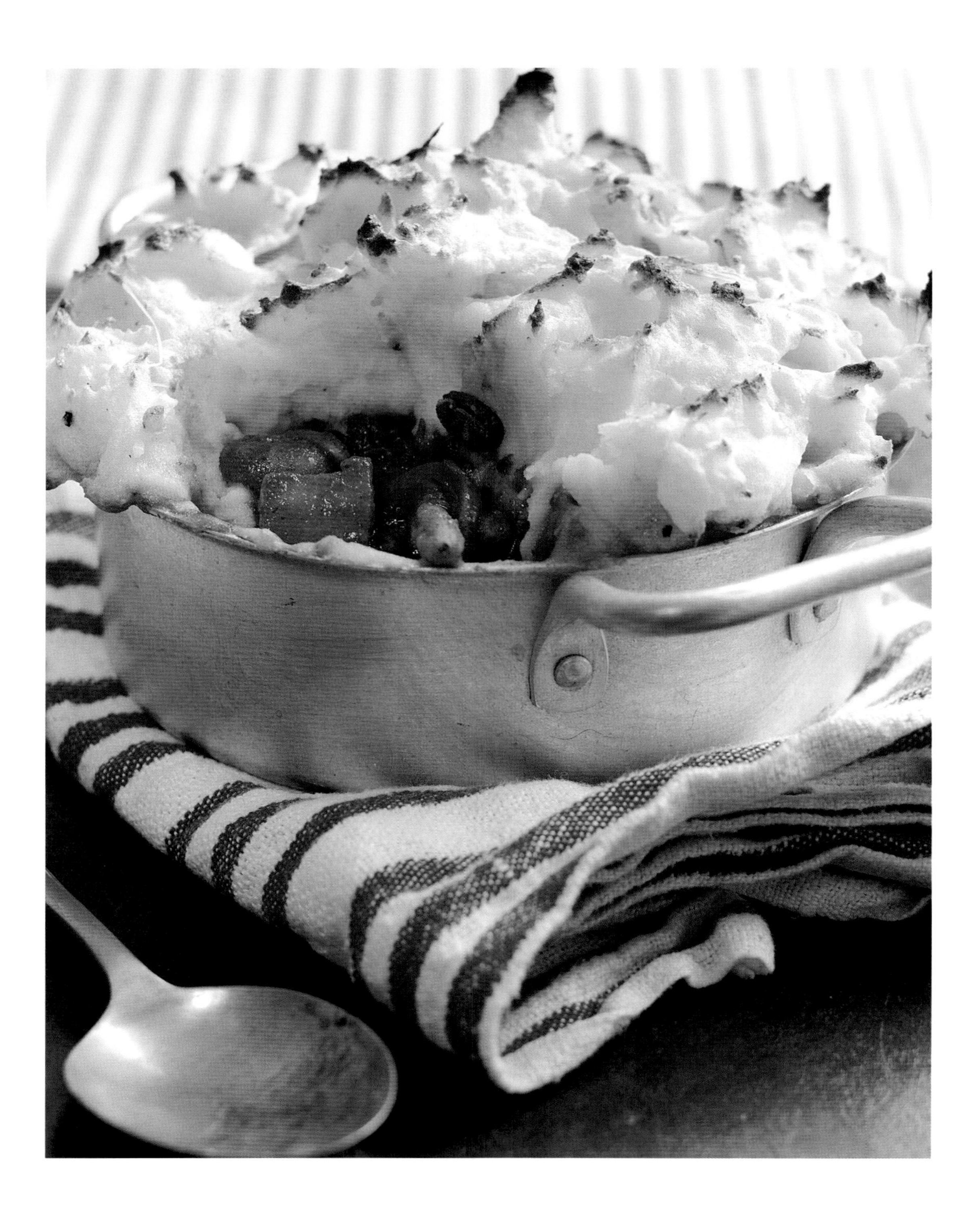

champion pie

Pie and mash is food for the soul: the best food to eat on a cold winter's day or when it's dull and raining, when it's guaranteed to make you feel better. Packed full of fibre, carbohydrates and iron, it will help flagging muscles recover quickly.

1 tablespoon olive oil
1 large onion, thinly sliced
2 teaspoons minced garlic
2 tablespoons red pesto
2 x 400 g cans of chopped tomatoes with herbs
300 ml (½ pint) vegetable stock
450 g (1 lb) butternut squash, peeled, seeded and cut into chunks
200 g (7 oz) fine green beans, trimmed
1 kg (2¼ lb) floury potatoes, such as Maris Piper, peeled and cut into chunks
150 ml (¼ pint) skimmed milk
1 bunch of spring onions, trimmed and shredded
410 g can of mixed pulses, drained and rinsed

Preparation: 25 minutes
Cooking time: 1½ hours
Serves 4

> Preheat the oven to 200°C/400°F/Gas Mark 6. Heat the oil in a large frying pan and fry the onion for 7–8 minutes over a low heat, until softened and golden. Add the garlic, red pesto, tomatoes, vegetable stock and butternut squash. Bring to the boil, cover and simmer for 15 minutes or until the butternut squash is tender.

> Meanwhile, blanch the green beans in lightly salted, boiling water for 3–4 minutes. Drain and refresh in cold water.

> Cook the potatoes in a large pan of lightly salted, boiling water for 10 minutes until tender. Tip into a colander to drain. Add the milk and spring onions to the pan and cook for 3–4 minutes, until the onions have softened. Tip the potatoes back into the pan and mash. Season to taste.

> Stir the green beans and pulses into the butternut squash mixture and transfer to a large ovenproof dish or four individual pie dishes. Spoon over the mash to cover and bake for 30–35 minutes, until golden.

nutritional information calories 404 • fat 6.5 g • saturated fat 1.3 g • added sugar none • fibre 13.2 g • protein 20.2 g • salt 1.31 g • carbohydrate 71 g

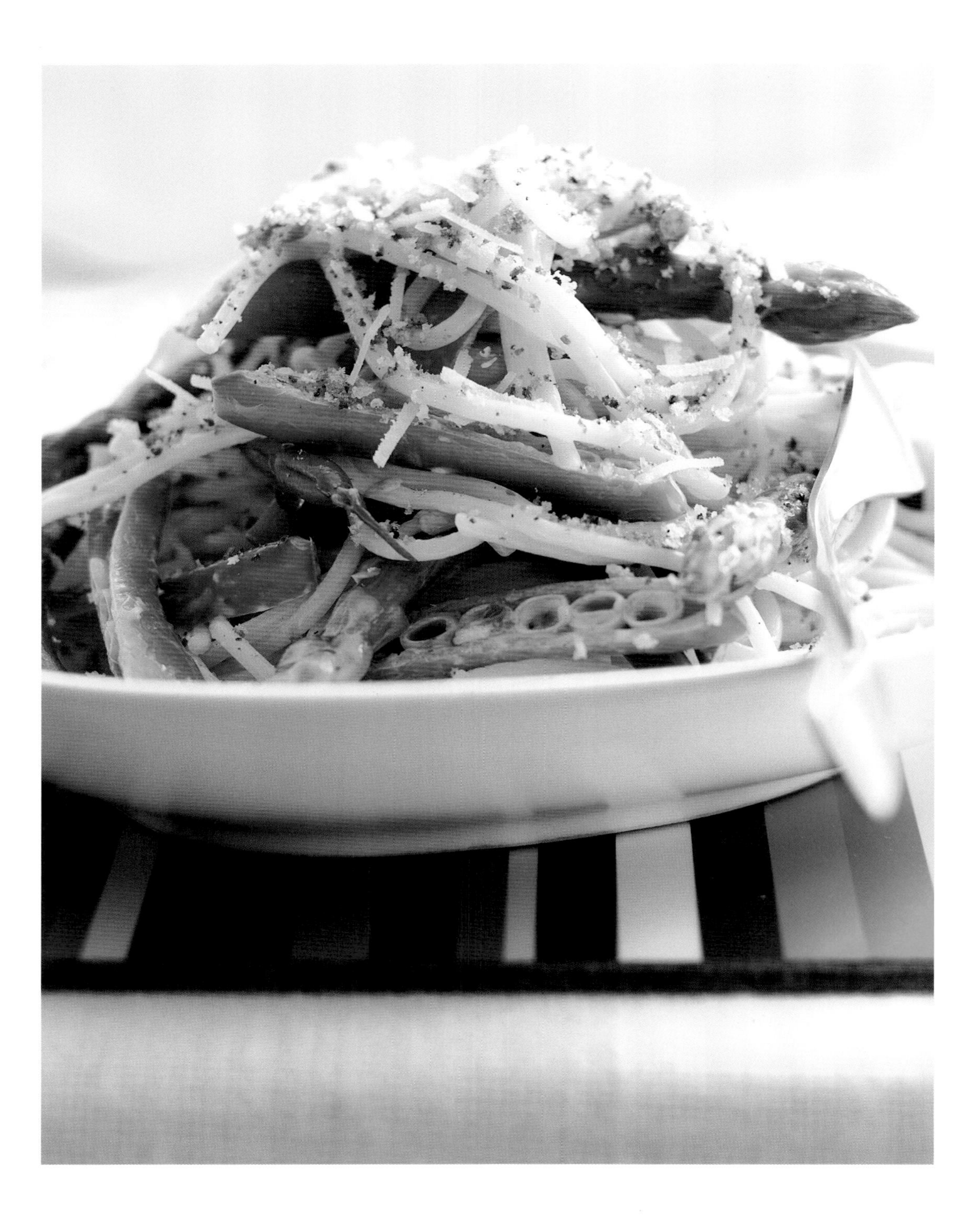

vitality pasta

This recipe shows that a little goes a long way: with a strongly flavoured cheese, such as the Parmesan used here, you need only a little to flavour the whole dish so the high fat content is not too problematic.

400 g (14 oz) spaghetti
1 bunch of asparagus spears, trimmed and halved
125 g (4 oz) fine green beans
200 g (7 oz) sugarsnap peas, trimmed and halved lengthways
2 teaspoons olive oil
2 garlic cloves, crushed
50 g (2 oz) white breadcrumbs
juice and finely grated zest of 1 large lemon
3 tablespoons half-fat crème fraîche
25 g (1 oz) Parmesan cheese, finely grated
salt and freshly ground black pepper

Preparation: 10 minutes
Cooking time: 13–15 minutes
Serves 4

> Cook the spaghetti in a large pan of lightly salted, boiling water for 8 minutes. Add the asparagus, fine green beans and sugarsnap peas, bring back to the boil and cook for 2–3 minutes.

> Meanwhile, heat the oil in a large frying pan and fry the garlic, breadcrumbs and lemon zest for 1–2 minutes, stirring until golden and crisp. Season with salt and pepper.

> Drain the pasta and vegetables and return to the hot pan. Stir in the crème fraîche, Parmesan cheese and lemon juice to taste. Season with salt and plenty of black pepper. Serve scattered with the crisp garlicky breadcrumbs.

nutritional information calories 485 • fat 7.8 g • saturated fat 2.8 g • added sugar none • fibre 5.3 g • protein 20 g • salt 0.71 g • carbohydrate 89 g

healthy eating

> Green vegetables taste best when cooked quickly so that they still have a crunch to them. This also means that you don't lose all their goodness in the cooking water.

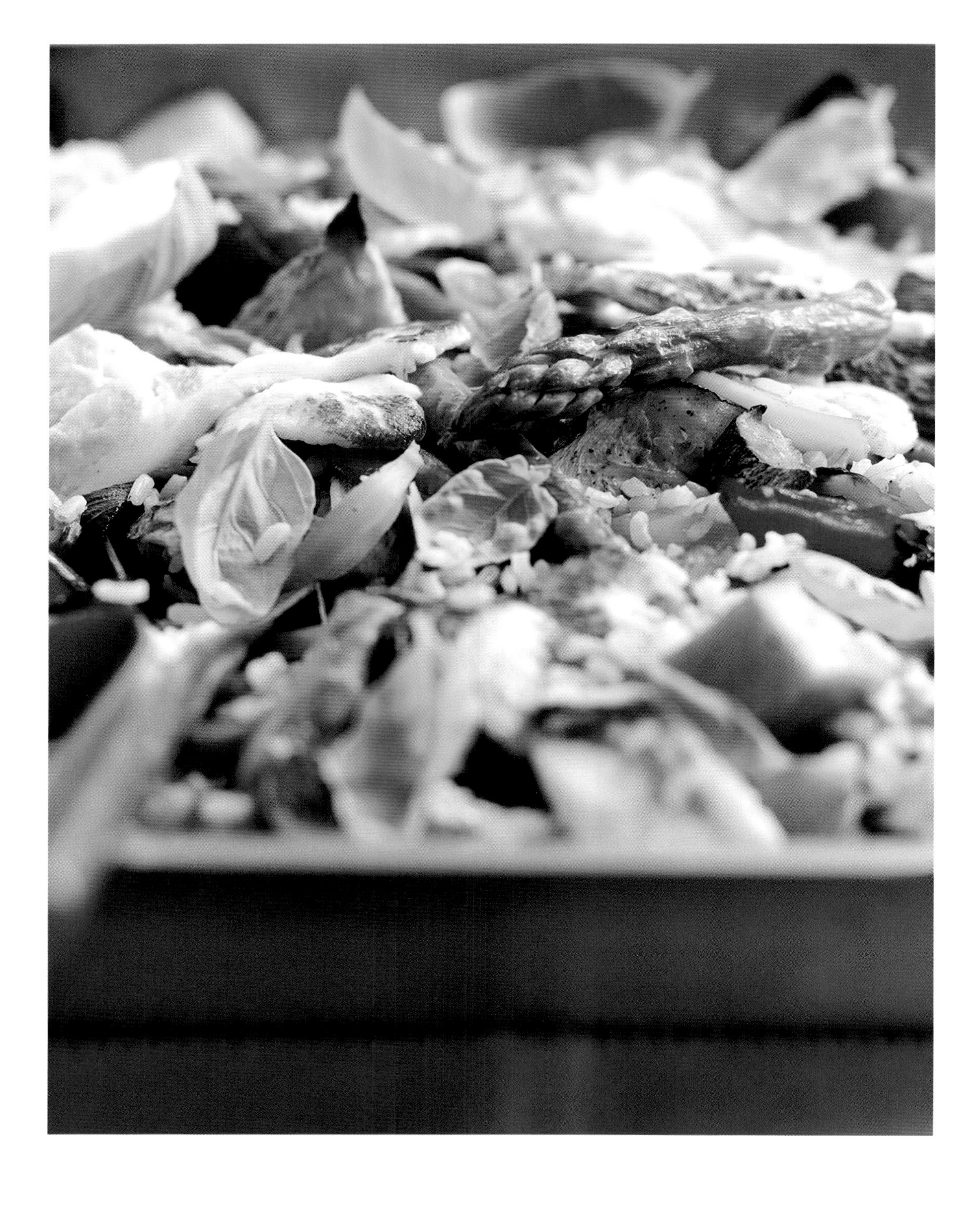

golden halloumi with roast vegetables

Many vegetables have their own natural sugars that, when roasted, turn into a sweet caramelised coating. Here roasted vegetables are tossed through brown rice and served with oozing golden halloumi cheese – what could be better?

2 large red onions, cut into wedges
1 large red pepper, seeded and cut into chunks
1 large orange or yellow pepper, seeded and cut into chunks
1 large brown-skinned, pink-fleshed sweet potato, peeled and cut into chunks
2 large carrots, peeled and sliced diagonally
1 large courgette, trimmed and cut into chunks
1 small whole head of garlic, cloves separated but unpeeled
2 tablespoons olive oil
125 g (4 oz) asparagus tips
2 tablespoons balsamic vinegar
225 g (8 oz) easy-cook brown rice
250 g (9 oz) halloumi cheese, cut into 8 thin slices
basil leaves, to garnish

Preparation: 20 minutes
Cooking time: 30 minutes
Serves 4

- Preheat the oven to 200°C/400°F/Gas Mark 6. Put the red onion, peppers, sweet potato, carrots, courgette, garlic and 1 tablespoon of the oil into a large roasting tin and toss together to coat. Roast for 20 minutes. Toss the asparagus tips and balsamic vinegar into the roasted vegetables and roast for a further 10 minutes.

- Meanwhile, cook the rice in a pan of lightly salted, boiling water, according to the packet instructions.

- About 6–8 minutes before the end of the cooking time, heat the remaining oil in a large frying pan and fry the halloumi cheese slices for 2–3 minutes on each side until golden. Remove from the pan and keep warm.

- Drain the rice. Remove the vegetables from the oven and pop the garlic cloves from their papery skins. Mash with a fork and stir into the rice, with the other roasted vegetables. Serve topped with the golden halloumi cheese and scatter with fresh basil leaves.

nutritional information calories 609 • fat 23.9 g • saturated fat 10.7 g • added sugar none • fibre 8.2 g • protein 21.6 g • salt 2.42g • carbohydrate 82 g

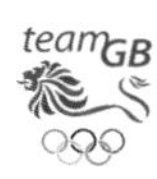

Colin Jackson's

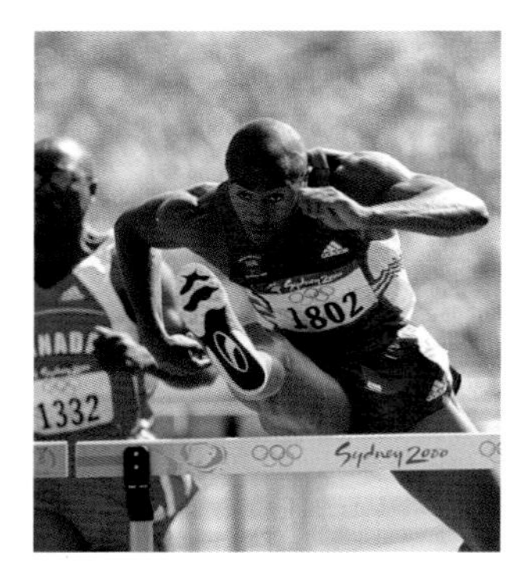

stir-fried bok choy with noodles

This recipe is great – not only is it good for me but it tastes good too. I often stir-fry some protein, such as prawns or chicken, and add it to the stir-fry with the mushrooms and bok choy.

25 g (1 oz) wholemeal angel-hair pasta or spaghetti
1 tablespoon soy sauce
1 tablespoon teriyaki sauce
2 tablespoons dry sherry
1 teaspoon minced ginger
2 teaspoons olive oil
125 g (4 oz) bok choy, sliced
125 g (4 oz) shiitake mushrooms, thickly sliced
2 spring onions, sliced

Preparation: 5–10 minutes
Cooking time: 10 minutes
Serves 1

> Cook the pasta in a pan of lightly salted, boiling water for 5 minutes. Drain well and set aside.

> Mix together the soy and teriyaki sauces, sherry and ginger in a small bowl.

> Heat the oil in a large frying pan or wok. Add the bok choy and mushrooms and stir-fry for 2 minutes. Pour over the sauce, add the pasta and stir-fry for a further 2 minutes. Add the spring onions, mix well and serve immediately.

nutritional information calories 219 • fat 7.2 g • saturated fat 1 g • added sugar 0.6 g • fibre 2.3 g • protein 8.5 g • salt 6.5 g • carbohydrate 23 g

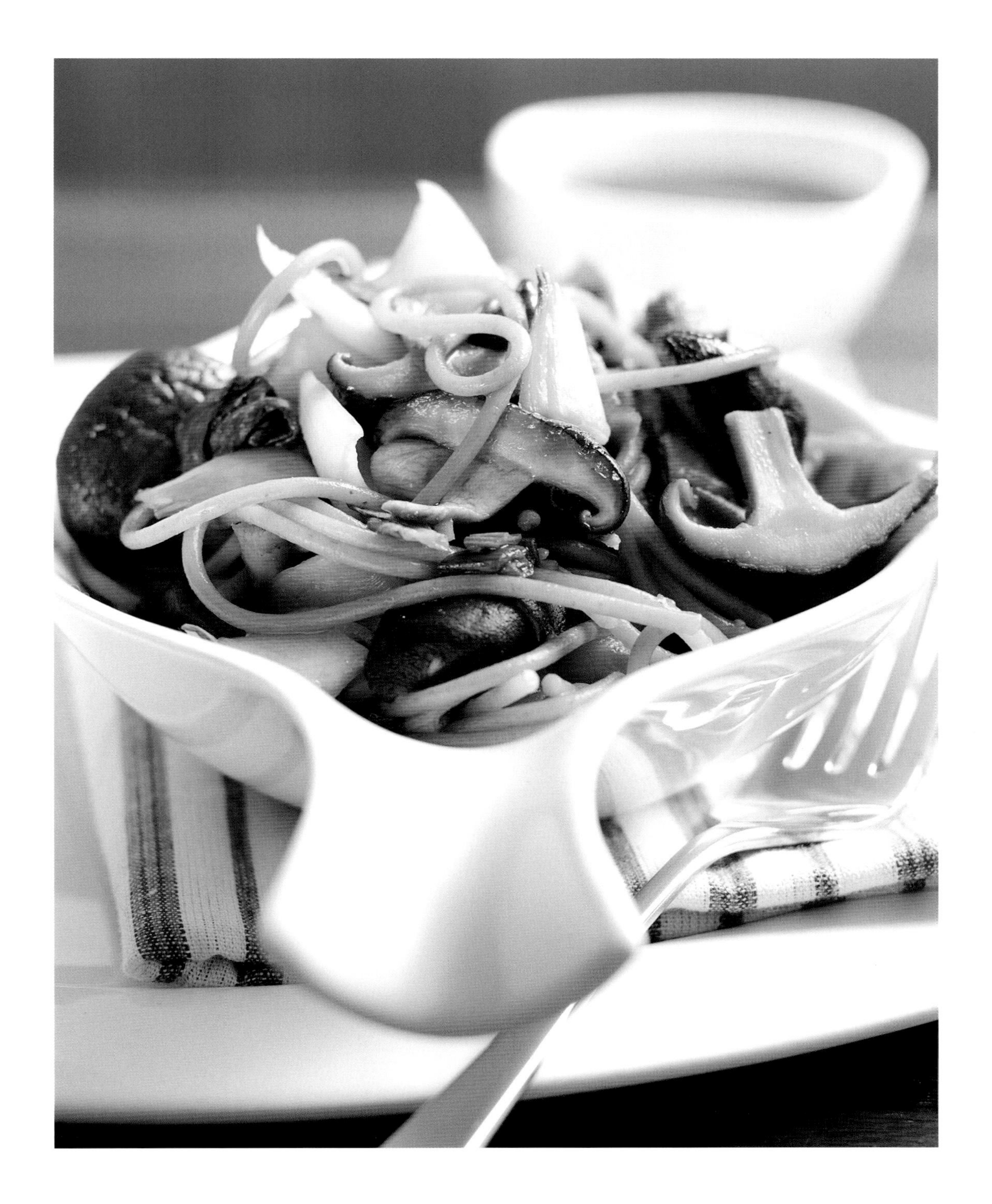

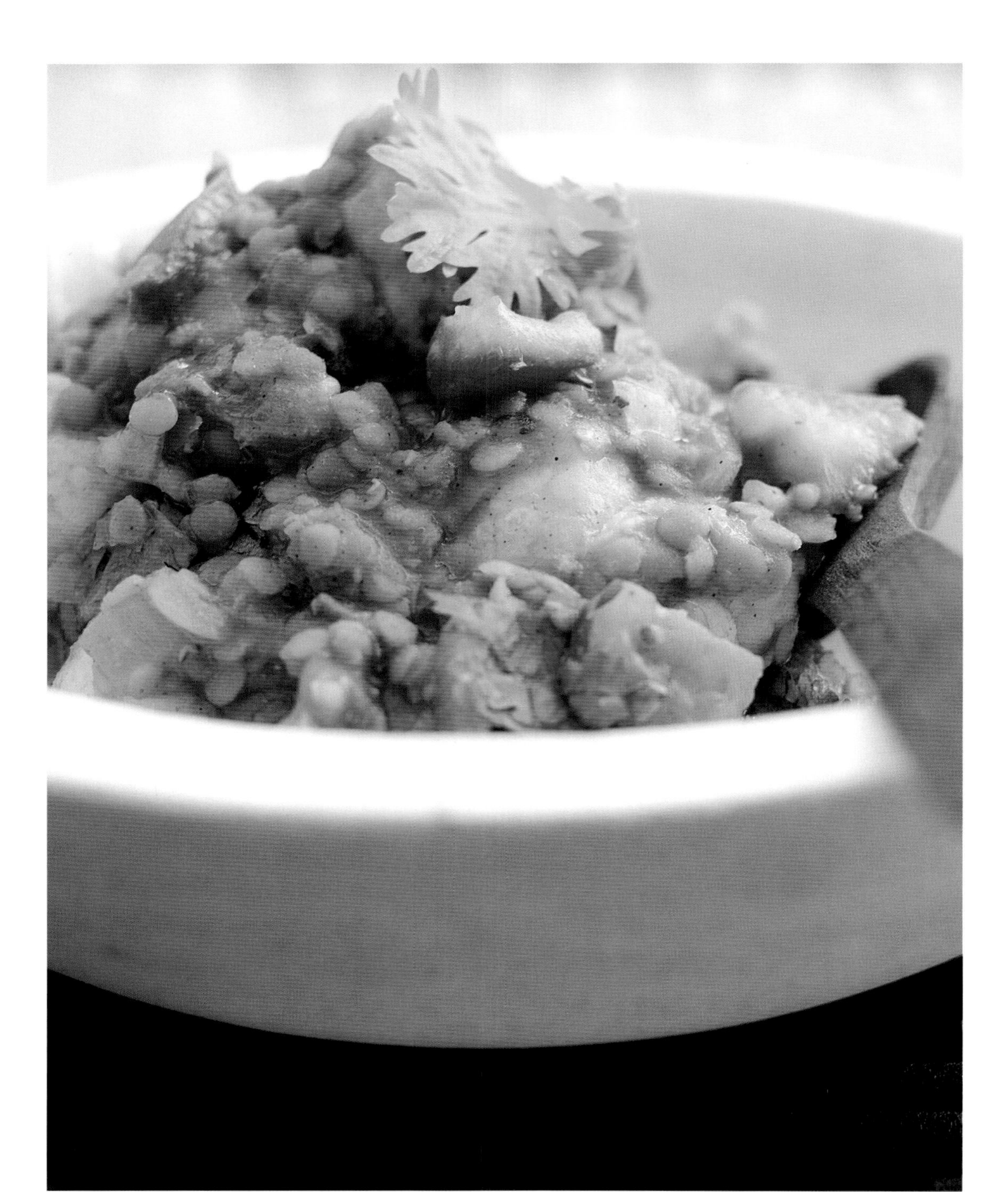

spicy tomato and cauliflower dhal

Lentils are a great source of zinc, protein and carbohydrate. I often cook this mixture and spoon it over warm naan breads or use red pesto to flavour it instead of the Indian spices, or top it with mashed potato for a really tasty veggie shepherd's pie.

800 g (1¾ lb) small cauliflower florets
1 tablespoon olive oil
2 onions, chopped
1 tablespoon garam masala
225 g (8 oz) red lentils
900 ml (1½ pints) vegetable stock
4 ripe tomatoes, roughly chopped
salt and freshly ground black pepper
small handful of chopped coriander leaves, to garnish

Preparation: 15 minutes
Cooking time: 40–45 minutes
Serves 4

> Cook the cauliflower florets in lightly salted, boiling water for 6–7 minutes, until just tender.

> Meanwhile, heat the oil in a large saucepan and fry the onions over a low heat for 7–8 minutes until softened and beginning to brown. Stir in the garam masala and cook for 1 minute, stirring. Add the lentils and stock. Bring to the boil, cover and cook for 20 minutes.

> Drain the cauliflower and stir into the lentils with the tomatoes. Simmer for 5–10 minutes until the lentils are tender. Season to taste and serve scattered with fresh coriander.

nutritional information calories 329 • fat 6.3 g • saturated fat 0.4 g • added sugar none • fibre 8.1 g • protein 23.6 g • salt 0.87 g • carbohydrate 47 g

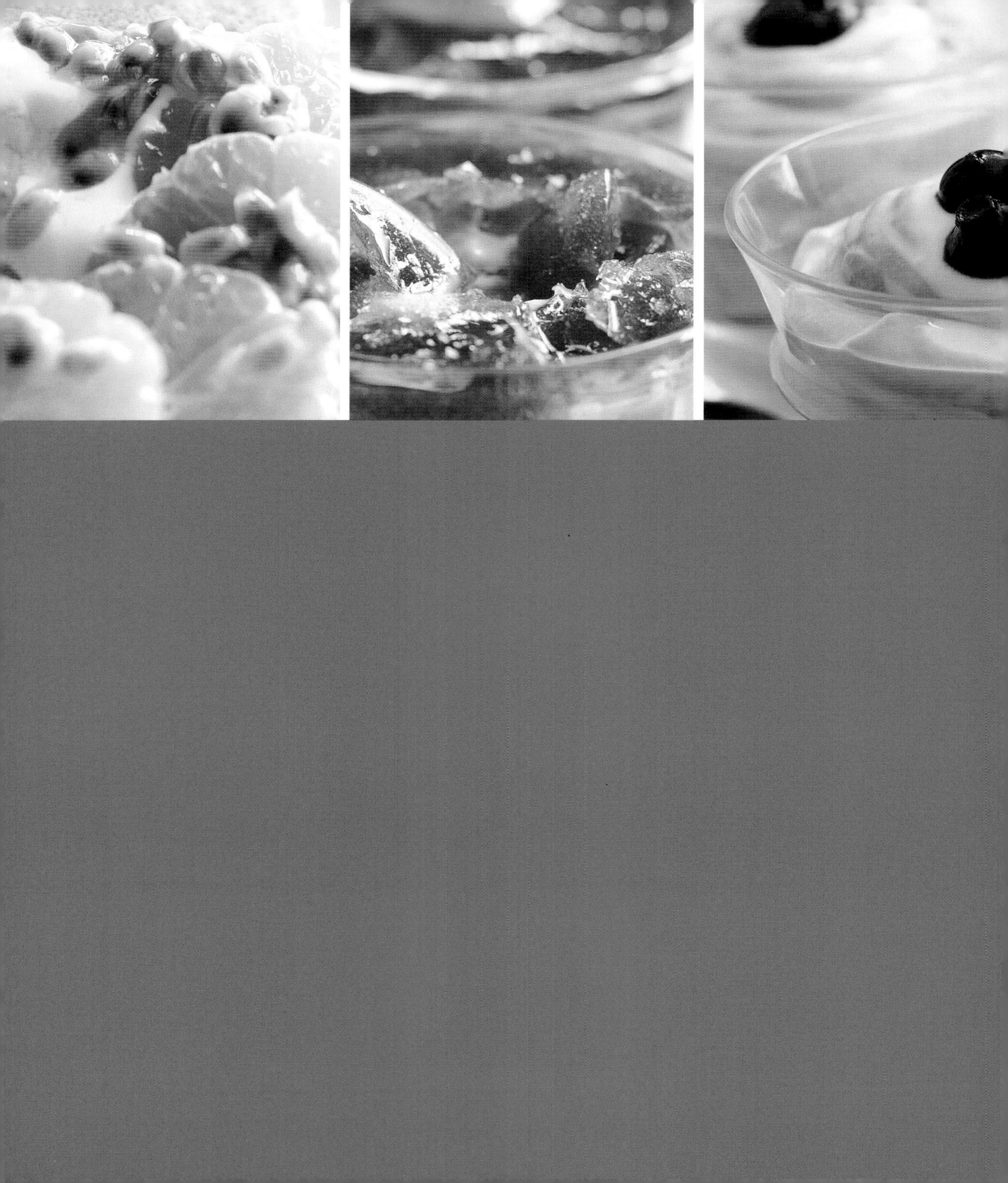

desserts

There are very few of us who can say, hand-on-heart, that we don't like dessert. Sometimes we all feel the need to indulge, and what better way to do it than with a bowlful of delicious creamy pud? Of course, if you're aiming to improve your diet, too many portions of roly-poly pudding are not a good thing, but you can still live a little. In the following pages you'll find a mouth-watering selection of creamy, fruity and comforting desserts that won't pile on the pounds.

Sally Gunnell's

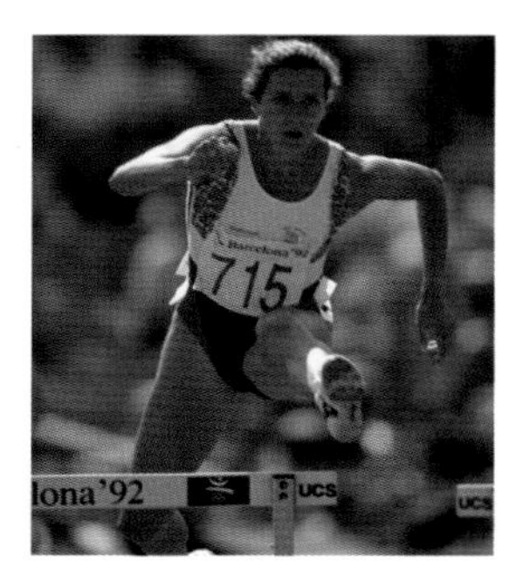

passion-fruit water ice

This is one of my favourite puddings: it's fresh and palate-tingingly sensational. A joy to eat and a delight to make – quick, easy and ready to go into the freezer in 20 minutes.

225 g (8 oz) caster sugar
8 passion-fruits
1 egg white

Preparation: 10 minutes
Cooking time: 15 minutes
Serves 4

> Put the caster sugar in a large, heavy-based saucepan with 600 ml (1 pint) water. Heat gently, stirring occasionally, until the sugar has dissolved. Bring to the boil and boil gently for 10 minutes. Leave to cool.

> Cut the passion-fruits in half. Scoop out the flesh and sieve to remove the seeds. Stir into the cooled sugar syrup and pour into a freezerproof container. Freeze for 2 hours until just beginning to freeze around the edges.

> Whisk the egg white until stiff. Remove the passion-fruit mixture from the freezer and stir with a fork to break up any large ice crystals. Fold in the whisked egg white and return to the freezer until ready to use. Remove from the freezer 15 minutes before serving. Spoon into glasses and serve immediately.

nutritional information calories 235 • fat 0.1 g • saturated fat none • added sugar 59.1 g • fibre 1 g • protein 1.5 g • salt 0.06 g • carbohydrate 61 g

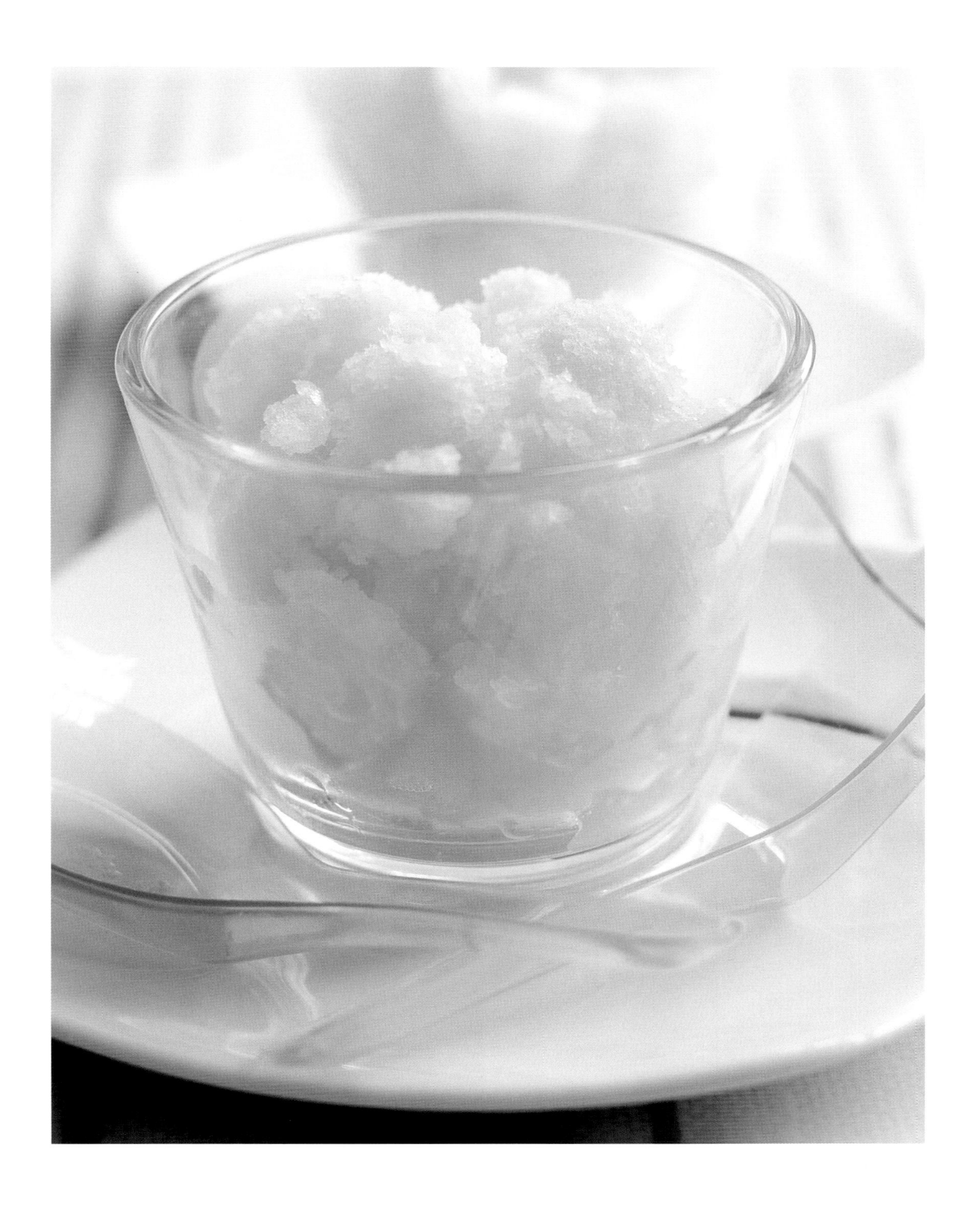

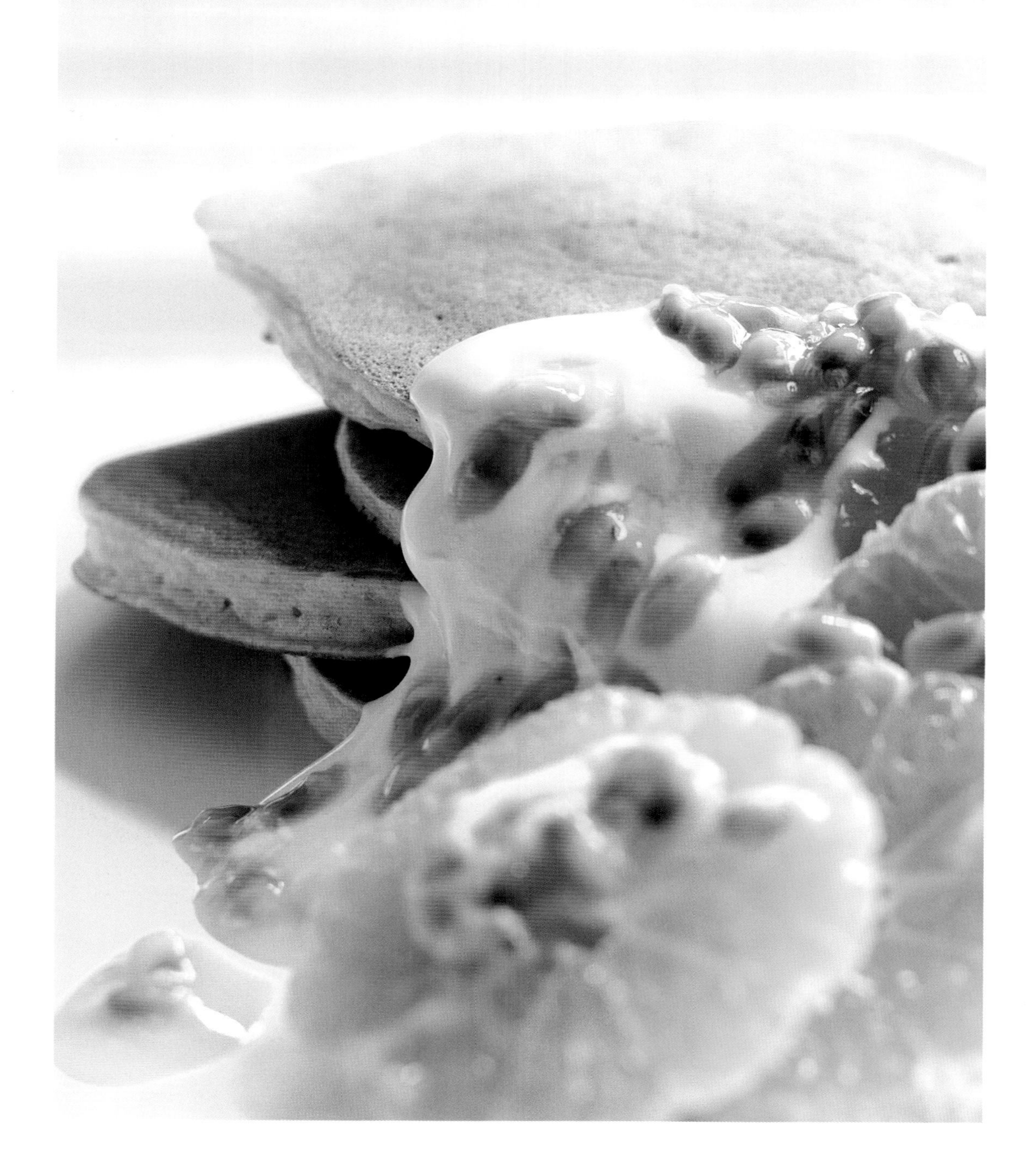

zesty st clement's pancakes

Serve these pancakes with a filling of your favourite fruits. They can be made up to 2 days in advance and then warmed through in the microwave or in a moderate oven for 5 minutes.

6 clementines
50 g (2 oz) caster sugar
100 ml (4 fl oz) fresh orange juice
250 g (9 oz) low-fat lemon yoghurt
1 medium egg
25 g (1 oz) butter, melted
150 g (5 oz) plain flour
1 teaspoon bicarbonate of soda
1 teaspoon baking powder
sunflower oil spray
2 passion-fruits, halved
6 tablespoons half-fat crème fraîche, to serve (optional)

Preparation: 15–20 minutes
Cooking time: 12–15 minutes
Serves 6

> Peel the clementines and remove as much pith as possible (although a little bit laborious, this is well worth the effort, but if you don't fancy this job, simply segment the clementines). Slice them horizontally.

> Whisk the caster sugar, 50 ml (2 fl oz) of the orange juice, the yoghurt, egg, butter, plain flour, bicarbonate of soda and baking powder together in a large bowl until smooth. Leave for 10 minutes to rest.

> Spray the bottom of a large non-stick frying pan with sunflower oil and put on to a medium heat. Drop 4 dessertspoons of the batter into the frying pan, equally spaced apart, and cook for 1–2 minutes on each side, or until golden. (When the top of the pancake is covered with tiny air bubbles, it's time to turn it over.) Set aside and keep warm while repeating to make 24 pancakes.

> Put the remaining orange juice and prepared clementines into a saucepan and squeeze in the passion-fruit seeds and juice. Warm through gently. Serve a stack of four pancakes per person with the clementine slices and the juices spooned over, and top each serving with a spoonful of half-fat crème fraîche, if liked.

nutritional information calories 229 • fat 5.4 g • saturated fat 2.7 g • added sugar 13.6 g • fibre 1.6 g • protein 5.7g • salt 1.02 g • carbohydrate 42 g

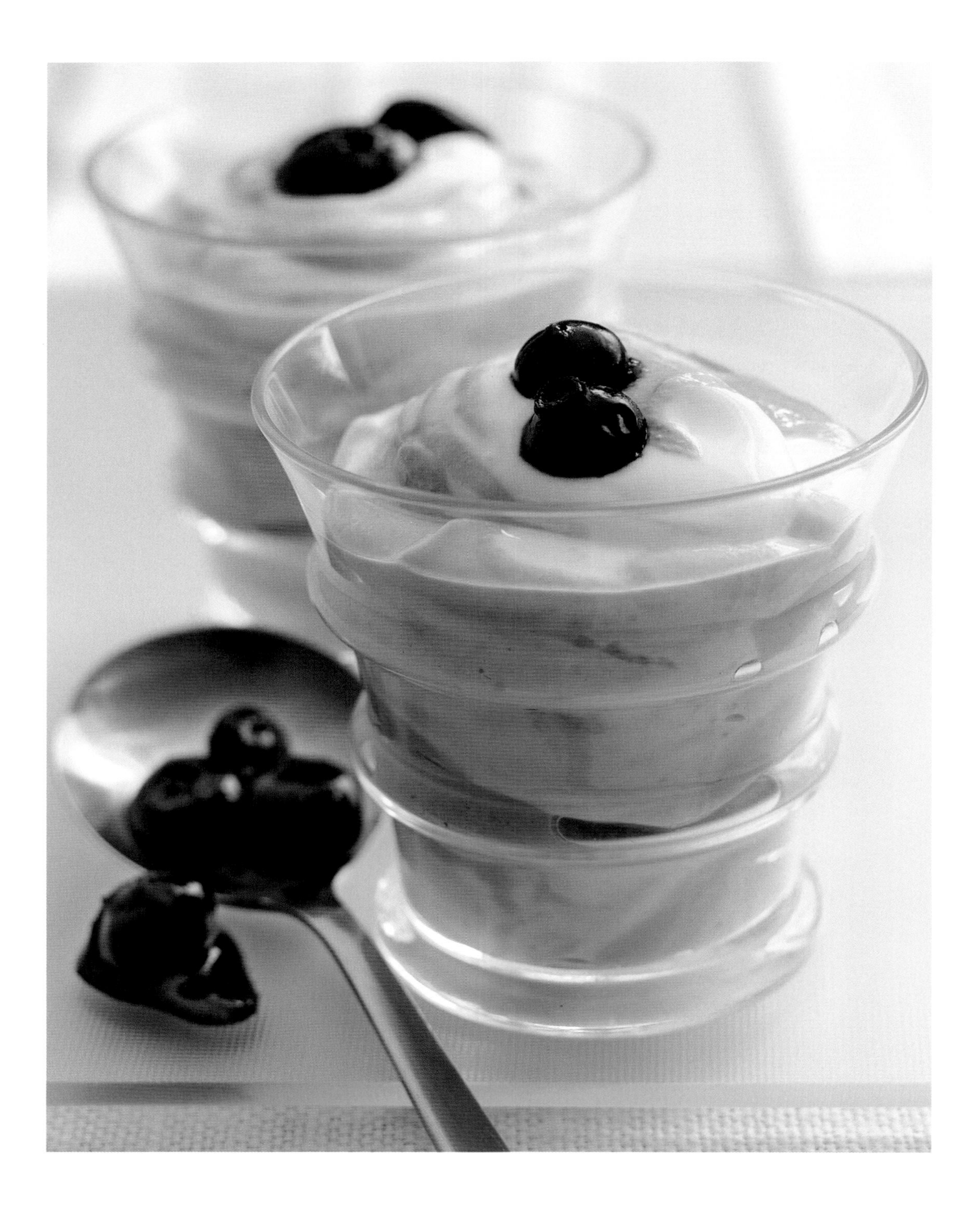

blueberry ripple

Simple, quick and only five ingredients – what could be better? I love the taste of blueberries, but you could also use blackberries, blackcurrants or raspberries for this dessert: simply sprinkle over a little more sugar if the berries are tart.

juice of 1 lime
150 g (5 oz) fresh blueberries
50 g (2 oz) caster sugar
2 x 250 g tubs of quark (skimmed-milk soft cheese)
200 ml tub of half-fat crème fraîche

Preparation: 10–15 minutes
Cooking time: 2–3 minutes
Serves 4

- Place the lime juice, blueberries and caster sugar in a pan. Heat gently, stirring occasionally, until the blueberries pop and release their juices. Leave to cool slightly.

- Reserve a couple of spoonfuls to serve and then push the remaining blueberries and juice through a sieve.

- Mix together the quark and sieved blueberries. Tip the crème fraîche on top and stir only once or twice to ripple through the blueberry mixture. Spoon into glasses and chill until ready to serve.

- Just before serving, spoon over the reserved blueberries.

nutritional information calories 237 • fat 7.6 g • saturated fat 4.7 g • added sugar 13.1 g • fibre 0.7 g • protein 20.3 g • salt 0.27 g • carbohydrate 23 g

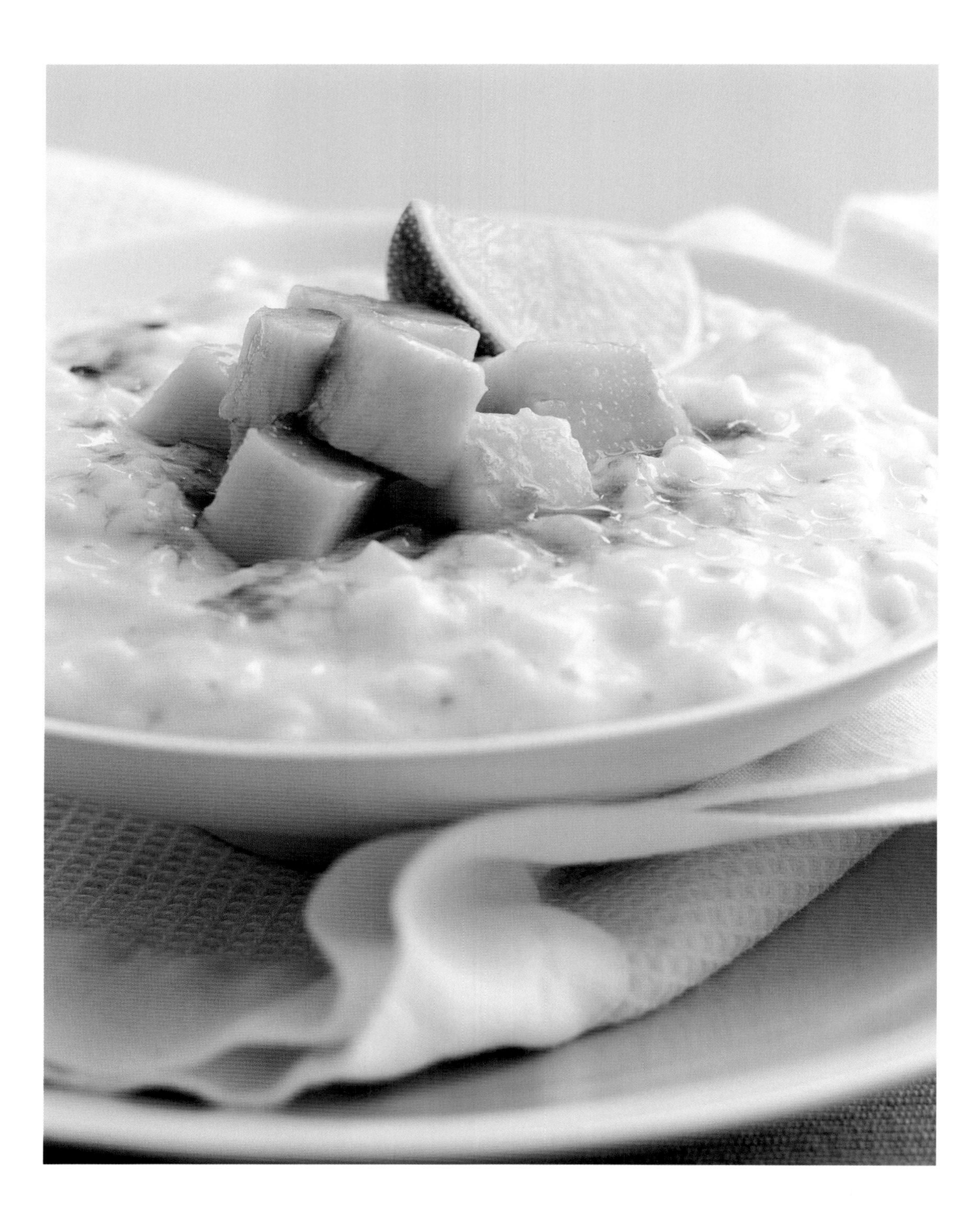

sweet rice pudding with mango and lime

Made using mostly storecupboard ingredients, this is a lower-fat version of the ultimate comfort food – how good is that? Served with mango it's all good for you and makes a great end to a relaxed weekend lunch.

175 g (6 oz) pudding rice
juice and finely grated zest of 2 limes
397 g can of sweetened condensed milk
1 large mango, peeled, stoned and cut into chunks
2 tablespoons soft light brown sugar
lime wedges, to serve (optional)

Preparation: 10 minutes
Cooking time: 30 minutes
Serves 4

> Place the rice, lime juice and zest and 850 ml (1½ pints) water in a large saucepan. Bring to the boil and simmer very gently, uncovered, for 25 minutes, stirring occasionally.

> Stir in the condensed milk and leave to cool slightly. Spoon into individual serving bowls. Spoon over the fresh mango chunks and sprinkle with brown sugar. Serve each portion topped with a lime wedge for squeezing over, if you wish.

nutritional information calories 540 • fat 10.9 g • saturated fat 6.3 g • added sugar 50.5 g • fibre 1.6 g • protein 12.6 g • salt 0.37 g • carbohydrate 104 g

healthy eating

> Mangoes are delicious and are bursting with antioxidants such as beta-carotene and vitamin C. To peel a mango, slice either side of the central stone, then cut lightly down and across each half to form a lattice pattern (ensuring that you don't cut through the skin). Turn each half inside out and scrape off the cubes of fruit into a bowl.

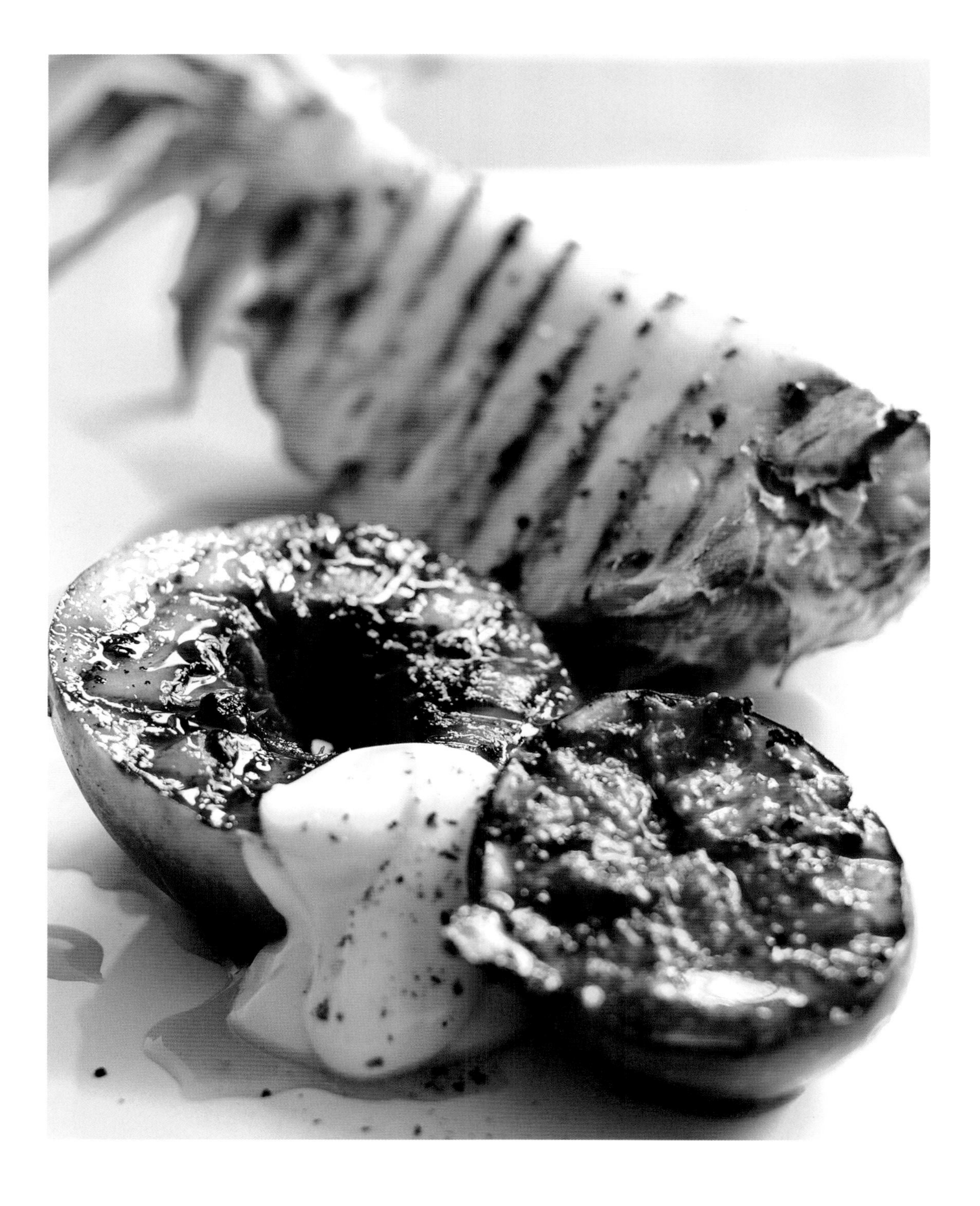

hot and sticky barbecued fruits

I love to barbecue everything, even fruits. Their natural sugars caramelise over the hot coals to create a great-tasting dessert. Black pepper and rum give this a spicy Jamaican flavour that is sure to get your tastebuds tingling.

2 tablespoons dark rum
juice of 1 lime
2 tablespoons runny honey
1 tablespoon freshly ground black pepper
1 small pineapple, quartered
2 nectarines, halved and stoned
2 figs, halved
4 tablespoons half-fat crème fraîche, to serve (optional)

Preparation : 15 minutes
Cooking time: 12–15 minutes
Serves 4

- Heat a large griddle pan until hot and smoking.
- Mix together the rum, lime juice, honey and black pepper. Toss the fruit in the rum mixture.
- Lay the pineapple on the griddle and cook for 5 minutes. Add the nectarines and figs, turn the pineapple over to the other side and cook for a further 5 minutes. Serve warm, with half-fat crème fraîche if you like, and any remaining sticky juices spooned over.

nutritional information calories 136 • fat 0.5 g • saturated fat none • added sugar 5.7 g • fibre 2.6 g • protein 2.1 g • salt 0.02 g • carbohydrate 29 g

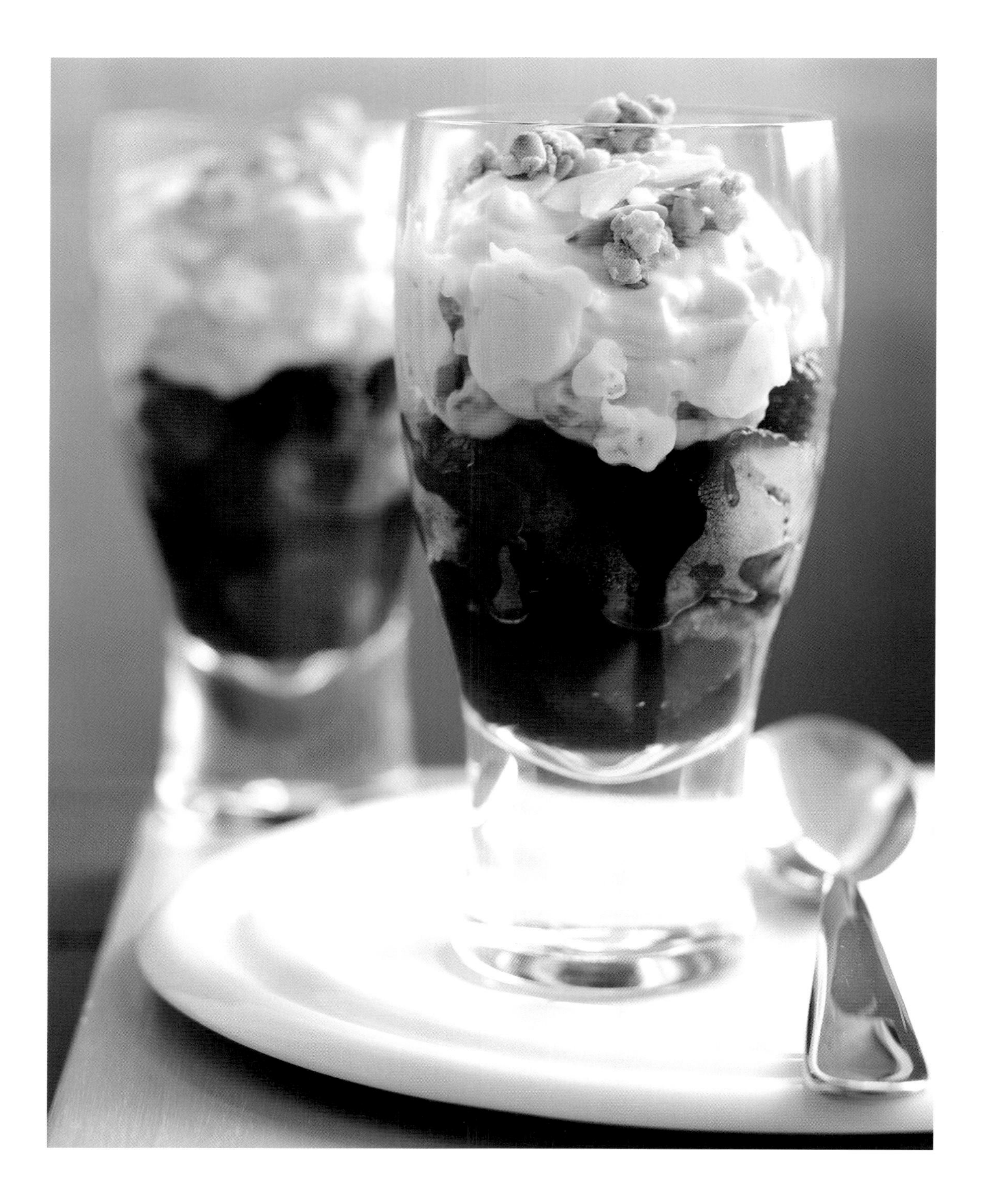

berry compote with honey crunch

There's a different texture in every mouthful of these irresistible desserts. The smooth, tangy berries and creamy, nutty yoghurt topped with sticky honey are a pure delight.

50 ml (2 fl oz) cranberry juice
1 large fresh mint sprig, plus extra leaves to decorate (optional)
450 g (1 lb) mixed berry fruit, such as strawberries, raspberries, blackberries and/or blueberries
2 x 200 g tubs of 0%-fat Greek-style yoghurt
2 tablespoons runny honey
50 g (2 oz) honey-nut cluster cereal
25 g (1 oz) toasted flaked almonds

Preparation: 10 minutes
Cooking time: 2 minutes
Serves 4

- Warm the cranberry juice and sprig of mint in a saucepan and stir in the fruit. Toss to coat evenly. Cover and set aside to cool completely. Discard the mint sprig.

- Mix together the Greek yoghurt and honey until smooth. Reserve a small handful of cereal and flaked almonds for decoration and then stir the remainder into the yoghurt mixture.

- Divide the fruit and juices between four glasses. Spoon over the yoghurt mixture and then sprinkle over the remaining cereal and the flaked almonds. Decorate with extra mint leaves if liked.

nutritional information calories 200 • fat 4.3 g • saturated fat 0.1 g • added sugar 10.2 g • fibre 3.1 g • protein 13.4 g • salt 0.44 g • carbohydrate 29 g

❛ Between my main meals I had to snack, so I'd fill up on cheese or beans on toast after school. ❜ >**Sharron Davies**

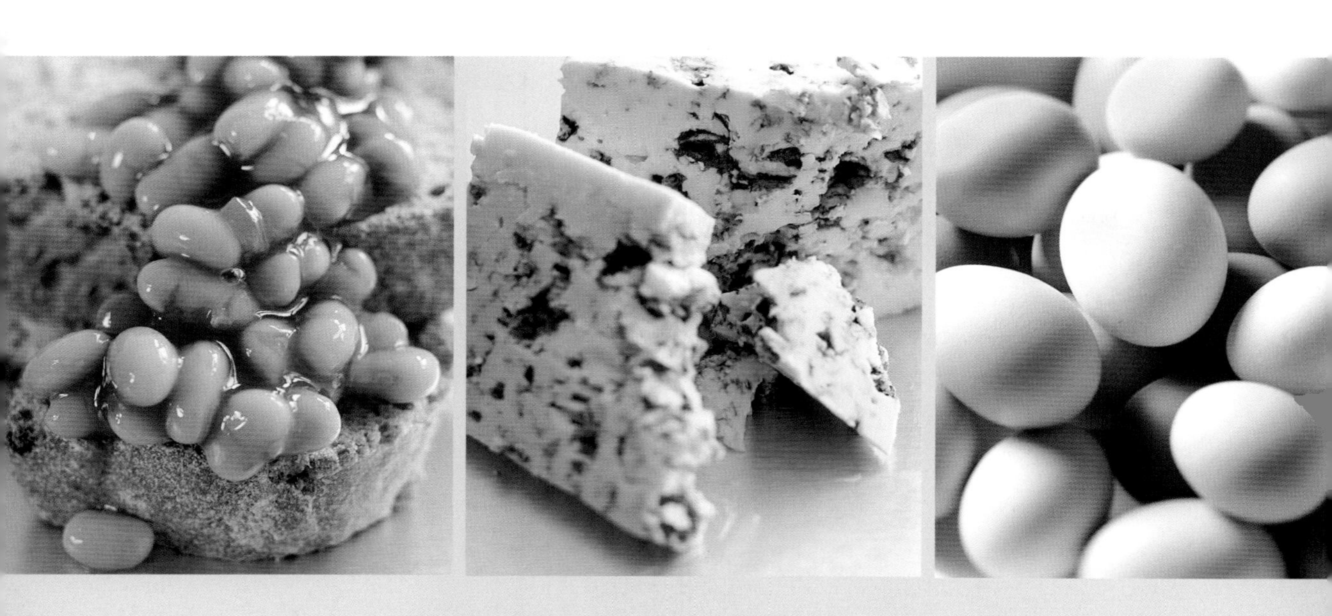

❛ Resuming my career as an adult meant that I had finished growing and didn't need as much food. ❜ >**Sharron Davies**

Success in swimming started early for Sharron Davies when, aged thirteen years and nine months, she became the youngest member of the British Team for the 1976 Montreal Olympics. As a growing teenager in serious training, it was vital that Sharron ate enough foods and in the correct balance to provide carbohydrate fuel for her muscles and nutrients such as protein for growth and repair.

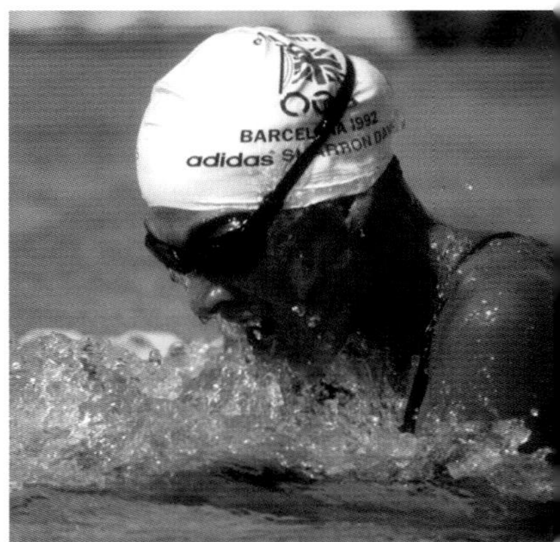

protein

The nutrients calcium, iron and zinc are needed in greater amounts by teenagers, yet many young people today eat a diet that falls short of their needs. Foods naturally high in calcium, iron and zinc also tend to be excellent sources of protein too: for example, milk, cheese and yoghurt contain plenty of calcium; red meat, poultry, eggs, nuts and dried beans are rich in zinc and iron. By eating enough of these foods the young Sharron Davies could prevent iron-deficiency anaemia and look after her immune system and her bones as well as providing the protein for muscle repair and growth. Sharron's diet was obviously exceptional, so how do we make sure that we get enough protein-rich foods in our diet? For good health we need to eat two to three portions of protein- and iron-rich foods every day. Each of the following represents a single portion:

- 50–125 g (2–4 oz) lean meat, poultry or fish
- 1–2 eggs
- 3 tablespoons dried beans or lentils

For calcium as well as protein, we all should be having three portions of milk and dairy foods daily, and teenagers probably need four! Examples of a portion could be 190 ml (⅓ pint) of semi or skimmed milk, a small tub of yoghurt, or a 25 g (1 oz) piece of cheese.

Sharron's food diary

> Breakfast

Bowl of muesli with milk – I never trained on an empty stomach – plus fruit juice, followed by a second breakfast after training of scrambled eggs on toast.

> Lunch

Chicken with potatoes and salad with some fruit and water.

> Main meal

I usually had two main evening meals – one before training and one on the way home after training! Before training I would eat something based around starchy carbohydrates like spaghetti bolognese and after training it was usually fish and chips as it saved mum cooking again!

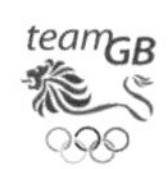

Ben Ainslie's oozing chocolate pots

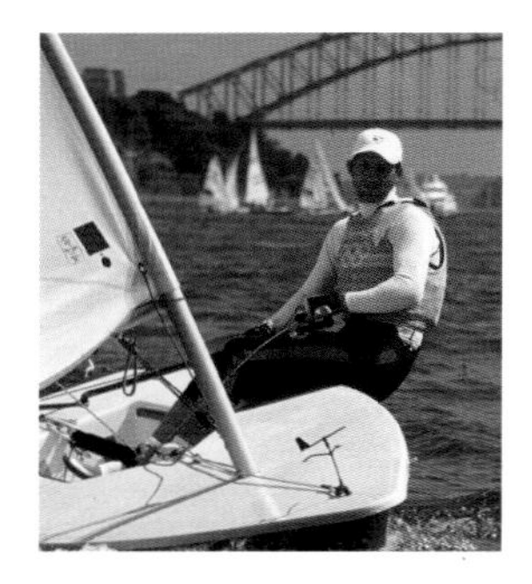

These easy chocolate soufflé puddings will be a real winner, whether you choose to make them for a special occasion or just as a treat. Don't do any guess work with the cooking time; it's the deciding factor as to whether you get the ooze or not!

60 g (2½ oz) unsalted butter
60 g (2½ oz) 70% dark chocolate
2 medium egg yolks
2 medium eggs
50 g (2 oz) caster sugar
50 g (2 oz) plain flour
icing sugar to dust

Preparation: 15–20 minutes
Cooking time: 15 minutes
Serves 4

> Preheat the oven to 180°C/350°F/Gas Mark 4. Melt the butter in a bowl set over a pan of simmering water. Use a small amount of the butter to very lightly grease the inside of 4 x 150 ml (¼ pint) ramekins, teacups or coffee cups.

> Add the chocolate to the remaining butter and heat until the chocolate has just melted. Whisk together the egg yolks, eggs and sugar using an electric whisk for about 4–5 minutes until thick, glossy and more than doubled in volume. Fold in the melted chocolate and plain flour until just mixed. Pour into the ramekins and bake for 12 minutes until risen but still soft to the touch. Dust with icing sugar to serve. If you are feeling brave you can turn out these little chocolate puddings: run a sharp knife around the inside edge of the ramekin and tip the pudding out onto your hand, then quickly pop it onto a plate. Serve with some fresh raspberries or ice cream.

nutritional information calories 360 • fat 24 g • saturated fat 12.5 g • added sugar 18.6 g • fibre 7.3 g • protein 6.9 g • salt 0.11 g • carbohydrate 31 g

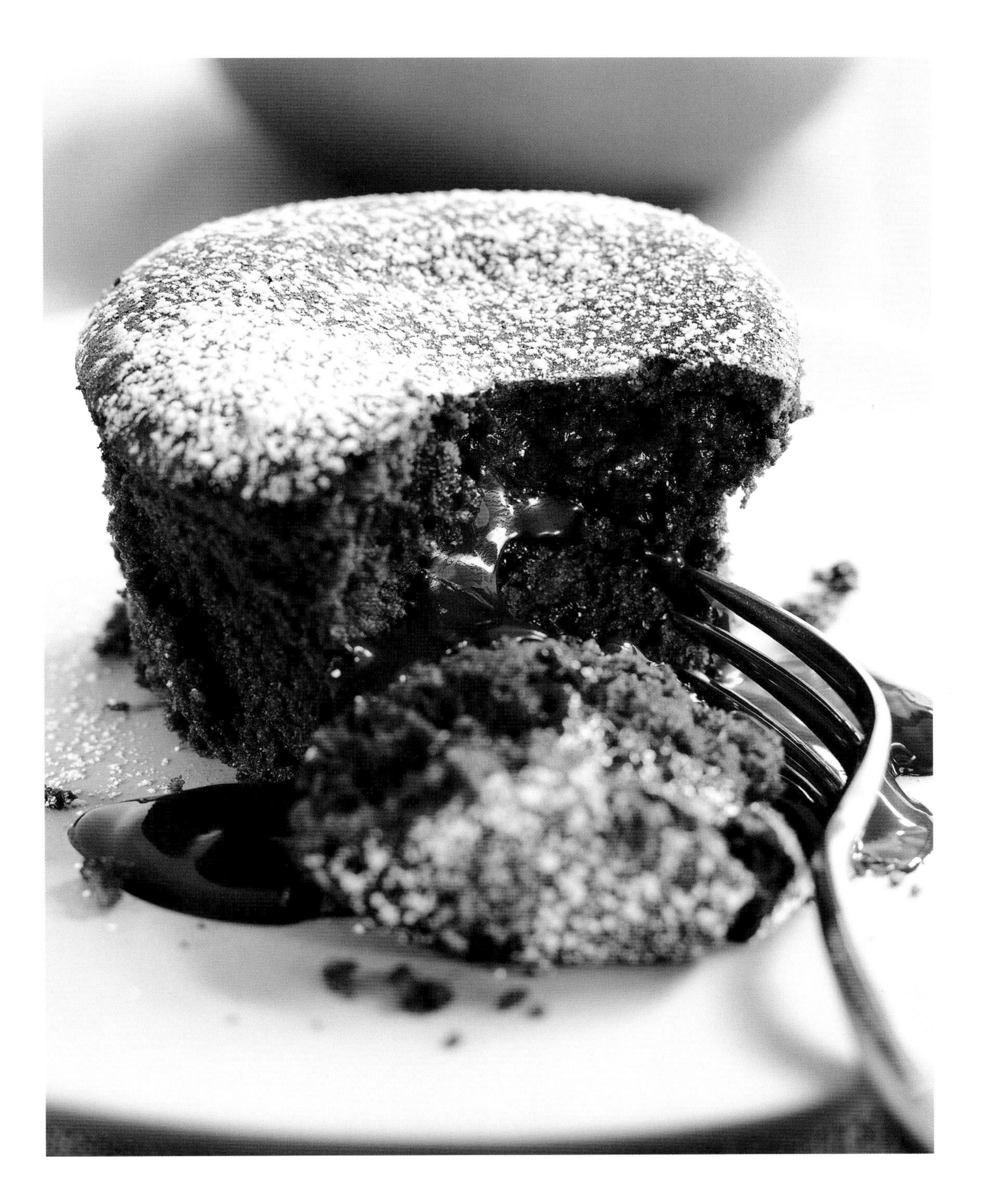

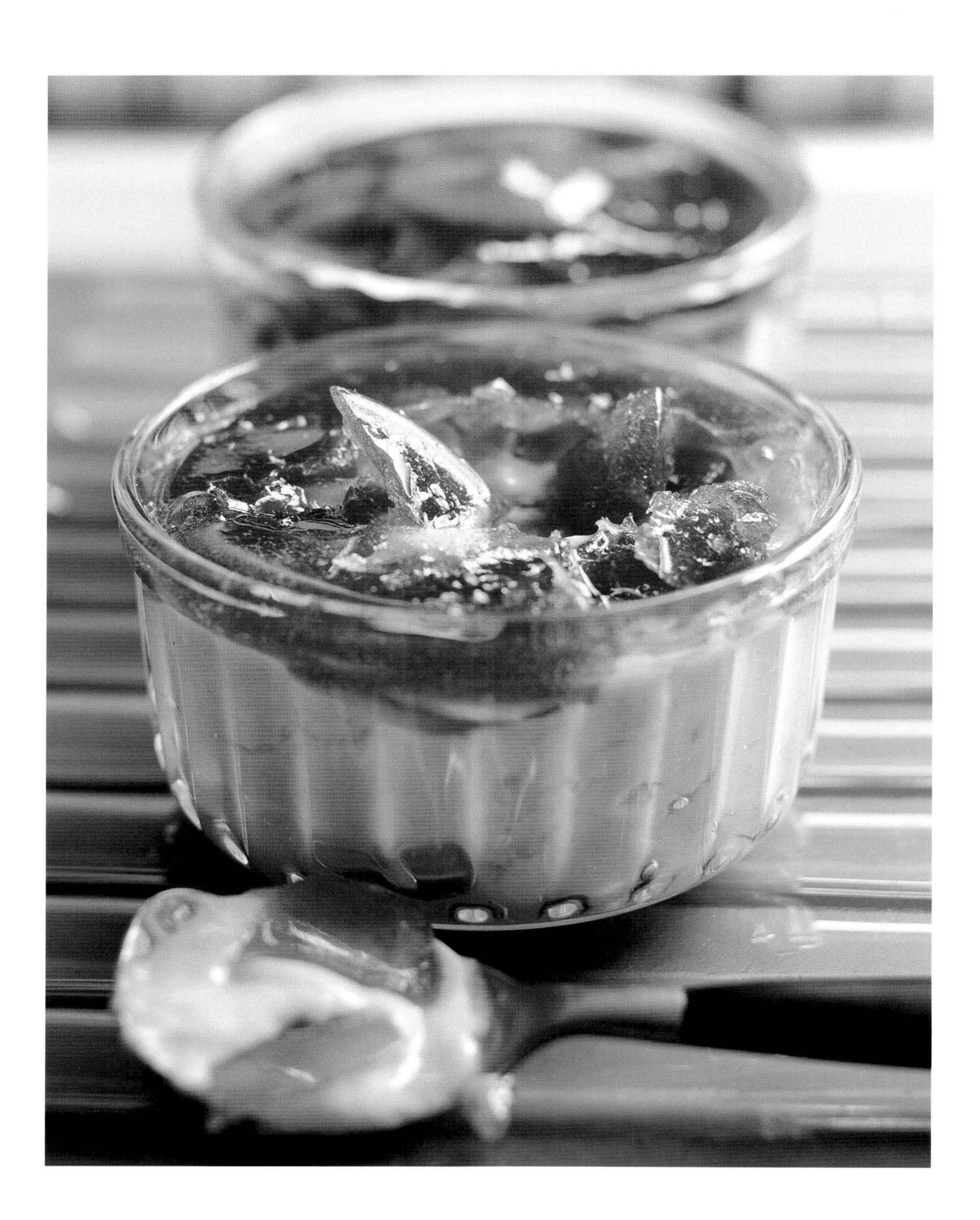

crackin' caramel and banana pots

Break through the caramel topping to reveal bananas and cream: what a cracking combination! This is banoffee pie without all the calories. It's sure to be a winner with the whole family.

2 large bananas
250 g tub of quark (skimmed-milk soft cheese)
2–3 tablespoons lemon curd
4 tablespoons half-fat crème fraîche
125 g (4 oz) caster sugar

Preparation time: 15 minutes
Cooking time: 2–3 minutes
Serves 4

> Mash one banana and stir in the quark, lemon curd and crème fraîche, until well combined. Then spoon into four 175 ml (6 fl oz) ovenproof glasses or ramekin dishes. Smooth the surface with the back of a spoon and chill for 15 minutes.

> Thinly slice the remaining banana and arrange over the top of the creamy mixture to cover. Sprinkle the sugar into a heavy-based pan and heat gently; cook until dissolved and golden brown. Be careful not to burn it. Quickly pour an equal amount of caramel over each ramekin, to cover the banana and creamy mixture. Leave to stand for 5 minutes to allow the sugar to set before serving immediately.

nutritional information calories 287 • fat 2.9 g • saturated fat 1.5 g • added sugar 35.5 g • fibre 0.8 g • protein 10.6 g • salt 0.13 g • carbohydrate 58 g

index

Ainslie, Ben, **11**, **124**
antioxidants, **7**, **29**
apples: fresh fruit muesli, **17**
apricots: energy bars, **35**
honeyed apricots with vanilla yoghurt, **18**
asparagus: vitality pasta, **101**

bagel, hot salmon, **25**
bananas: blue ribbon smoothie, **15**
crackin' caramel and banana pots, **127**
beans: champion pie, **99**
chicken with rice and peas, **70**
fire 'n' ice tortillas, **75**
saucy turkey chilli, **73**
spicy beans on toast, **97**
beef: sizzling beef in black bean stir-fry, **83**
steak sandwich with mustard sauce, **52**
berry compote with honey crunch, **121**
black bean stir-fry, sizzling beef in, **83**
blueberries: blue ribbon smoothie, **15**
blueberry ripple, **115**
bok choy stir-fried with noodles, **104**
bread: bacon-buster sarnie, **22**
hot and creamy prawns on toast, **59**
spicy beans on toast, **97**
steak sandwich with mustard sauce, **52**
breakfast, **12–35**
butterbeans: fresh tuna with gremolata butterbean salad, **87**
butternut squash: champion pie, **99**

calcium, **123**
caramel and banana pots, **127**
carbohydrates, **6**, **7**, **8–9**, **48–9**
carrots: energy in a glass, **15**
cauliflower: spicy tomato and cauliflower dhal, **107**
champion pie, **99**
cheese: golden halloumi with roast vegetables, **103**
see also quark
chick-peas: spicy beans on toast, **97**
sweet potato and chick-pea soup, **39**
chicken: chicken and ham carbonara, **68**
chicken caesar salad, **42**
chicken, pepper and pasta pot, **66**
chicken salad wraps, **55**
chicken with rice and peas, **70**
hot 'n' spicy Thai chicken and prawn salad, **47**
spiced chicken with raita couscous, **65**
yakitori chicken with udon vegetable noodles, **63**
chocolate: oozing chocolate pots, **124–5**

Christie, Linford, **10**, **70**, **94–5**
coconut baked fish with papaya and lime salsa, **85**
cod: coconut baked fish with papaya and lime salsa, **85**
couscous: spiced chicken with raita couscous, **65**

Davies, Sharron, **11**, **42**, **122–3**
desserts, **108–27**

Edwards, Jonathan, **10**, **78**
eggs: pepper and egg sauté, **21**
potato, rocket and tomato frittata, **33**
energy bars, **35**
energy in a glass, **15**

fats, **6**, **94–5**
figgy muffins, **31**
fire 'n' ice tortillas, **75**
five-spice pork, **77**
fluid intake, **7**
frittata, potato, rocket and tomato, **33**
fruit, **29**
berry compote with honey crunch, **121**
hot and sticky barbecued fruits, **119**
see also individual types of fruit

Gunnell, Sally, **11**, **110**

haddock *see* smoked haddock
ham: chicken and ham carbonara, **68**
Harland, Georgina, **11**, **28–9**, **56**
Harrison, Audley, **10**, **52**
honeyed apricots with vanilla yoghurt, **18**

immune system, **7**
iron, **123**

Jackson, Colin, **11**, **104**

kedgeree, one-pan, one-cook, **27**

lamb: kickin' lamb burgers with houmous, **81**
Moroccan lamb, **78**
lemon: zesty St Clement's pancakes, **113**
lentils: crunchy Puy lentil salad, **51**
spicy tomato and cauliflower dhal, **107**
lunch, **36–59**

mackerel *see* smoked mackerel
mango and lime, sweet rice pudding with, **117**
Mediterranean swordfish steaks, **91**
minerals, **7**, **28–9**, **123**
Moroccan lamb, **78**
muesli, fresh fruit, **17**

muffins, figgy, **31**
mussels in a bag, **93**

Niçoise salad, **56**
noodles: soba noodle broth with spring greens, **41**
speedy prawn and chilli stir-fry, **89**
stir-fried bok choy with, **104**
yakitori chicken with udon vegetable noodles, **63**

oats: energy bars, **35**
fresh fruit muesli, **17**
oils, **94–5**
orange: zesty St Clement's pancakes, **113**

pancakes, zesty St Clement's, **113**
papaya and lime salsa, coconut baked fish with, **85**
passion-fruit water ice, **110**
pasta: chicken and ham carbonara, **68**
chicken, pepper and pasta pot, **66**
stir-fried bok choy with noodles, **104**
vitality pasta, **101**
peas: one-pan, one-cook kedgeree, **27**
pepper and egg sauté, **21**
Pinsent, Matthew, **10**, **22**
pork: fire 'n' ice tortillas, **75**
five-spice pork, **77**
portion sizes, **6**
potatoes: champion pie, **99**
new potato, smoked mackerel and beetroot salad, **45**
potato, rocket and tomato frittata, **33**
prawns: hot and creamy prawns on toast, **59**
hot 'n' spicy Thai chicken and prawn salad, **47**
speedy prawn and chilli stir-fry, **89**
protein, **122–3**

quark: blueberry ripple, **115**
crackin' caramel and banana pots, **127**
hot salmon bagel, **25**

red kidney beans *see* beans
Redgrave, Sir Steve, **11**, **48–9**, **68**
rice: chicken with peas and, **70**
five-spice pork, **77**
golden halloumi with roast vegetables, **103**
one-pan, one-cook kedgeree, **27**
sweet rice pudding with mango and lime, **117**
rocket: potato, rocket and tomato frittata, **33**

salads: chicken caesar salad, **42**
chicken salad wraps, **55**
crunchy Puy lentil salad, **51**
fresh tuna with gremolata butterbean salad, **87**
hot 'n' spicy Thai chicken and prawn salad, **47**
new potato, smoked mackerel and beetroot salad, **45**
Niçoise salad, **56**
salmon *see* smoked salmon
seeds: energy bars, **35**
smoked haddock: one-pan, one-cook kedgeree, **27**
smoked mackerel: new potato, smoked mackerel and beetroot salad, **45**
smoked salmon: hot salmon bagel, **25**
smoothies, **15**
snacks, **7**
soba noodle broth with spring greens, **41**
soups: soba noodle broth with spring greens, **41**
sweet potato and chick-pea soup, **39**
spring greens, soba noodle broth with, **41**
superfoods, **28–9**
sweet potato and chick-pea soup, **39**
swordfish steaks, Mediterranean, **91**

tomatoes: potato, rocket and tomato frittata, **33**
saucy turkey chilli, **73**
spicy tomato and cauliflower dhal, **107**
tortillas: chicken salad wraps, **55**
fire 'n' ice tortillas, **75**
tuna: fresh tuna with gremolata butterbean salad, **87**
Niçoise salad, **56**
turkey: bacon-buster sarnie, **22**
saucy turkey chilli, **73**

vegetables, **29**
golden halloumi with roast vegetables, **103**
sizzling beef in black bean stir-fry, **83**
see also individual types of vegetable
vitality pasta, **101**
vitamins, **7**, **28–9**

water ice, passion-fruit, **110**

yoghurt: berry compote with honey crunch, **121**
fresh fruit muesli, **17**
honeyed apricots with vanilla yoghurt, **18**
spiced chicken with raita couscous, **65**

zinc, **123**